PAMELA STEPHEN

CW00370313

CHURCHILL LIVINGSTONE NURSING TEXTS

Nutrition and Dietetics for Nurses
Sixth edition
Mary E. Beck

Principles of Infection and Immunity in Patient Care
Caroline Blackwell and D. M. Weir

Practical Therapeutics for Nursing and Related Professions
Third edition
James A. Boyle

Practical Notes on Nursing Procedures
Seventh edition
J. D. Britten

**Norris and Campbell's Nurse's
Guide to Anaesthetics, Resuscitation
and Intensive Care**
Seventh edition
Donald Campbell and Alastair A. Spence

Drugs and Pharmacology for Nurses
Seventh edition
S. J. Hopkins

Essentials of Paediatrics for Nurses
Fifth edition
I. Kessel

Psychology as Applied to Nursing
Seventh edition
Andrew McGhie

Anatomy and Physiology Applied to Nursing
Fifth edition
Janet T. E. Riddle

Principles of Nursing
Third edition
Nancy Roper

Foundations of Nursing and First Aid
Fifth edition
Janet S. Ross and Kathleen J. W. Wilson

Bacteriology and Immunity for Nurses

Ronald Hare
MD

Emeritus Professor of Bacteriology in the University of London and formerly Honorary Consulting Bacteriologist to St Thomas's Hospital
Sometime Research Associate in the Connaught Medical Research Laboratories and Lecturer on Viruses, Hygiene and Preventive Medicine, University of Toronto

E. Mary Cooke
BSc, MD, FRCPath

Director, Division of Hospital Infection, Central Public Health Laboratory, London
Formerly Professor of Clinical Microbiology in the University of Leeds and Honorary Consultant in Clinical Microbiology to the Leeds Health Authority
Formerly Senior Lecturer and Honorary Consultant Bacteriologist, St Bartholomew's Hospital

SIXTH EDITION

Churchill Livingstone

EDINBURGH   LONDON   MELBOURNE AND NEW YORK   1984

CHURCHILL LIVINGSTONE
Medical Division of Longman Group Limited

Distributed in the United States of America by Churchill Livingstone Inc., 1560 Broadway,
New York, N.Y. 10036, and by associated companies, branches and representatives
throughout the world.

© Ronald Hare 1961, 1967
© Longman Group Limited 1972, 1975, 1979, 1984

All rights reserved. No part of this publication may be reproduced, stored in a retrieval
system, or transmitted in any form or by any means, electronic, mechanical,
photocopying, recording or otherwise, without the prior permission of the publishers
(Churchill Livingstone, Robert Stevenson House, 1–3 Baxter's Place, Leith Walk,
Edinburgh EH1 3AF).

First edition 1961
Second edition 1967
Third edition 1972
Fourth edition 1975
Fifth edition 1979
Sixth edition 1984

ISBN 0 443 02878 8

British Library Cataloguing in Publication Data
Hare, Ronald
    Bacteriology and immunity for nurses — 6th ed.
    1. Medical microbiology
    I. Title   II. Cooke, E. Mary
    616' 01'024613   QR46

Library of Congress Cataloging in Publication Data
Hare, Ronald.
    Bacteriology and immunity for nurses.
    (Churchill Livingstone nursing texts)
(Churchill Livingstone medical text)
    Includes index.
    1. Medical microbiology. 2. Communicable diseases — Prevention. 3. Immunology.
4. Nursing. I. Cooke, Edith Mary. II. Title. III. Series. IV. Series: Churchill Livingstone
medical text. [DNLM: 1. Bacteriology—Nursing texts. 2. Allergy and
immunology—Nursing texts. QW 4 H275b]
QR46.H29   1983   616'.01'024613   83-5314
ISBN 0-443-02878-8

Printed in Singapore by
Selector Printing Co (Pte) Ltd.

Preface

In the four years that have elapsed since the preparation of the previous edition new developments have occurred which have necessitated changes in the text. These include the addition of short sections on Legionnaire's disease, campylobacter infections and clostridial colitis. The section on antibiotics has been expanded in response to an increasing interest by nurses in antibiotic therapy. However, smallpox is now accorded only a brief mention. There has also been some rearrangement of the contents of the final chapters, resulting in an additional chapter.

We have continued to place the major emphasis of the book on the prevention of infection, reflecting the importance of nurses in this as part of their normal activities, as well as their increasing involvement as infection control nurses.

We have also continued to describe some techniques which are not used in modern hospitals, as we are aware that nurses may work under conditions very different from those which exist in developed countries. We have paid attention as in previous editions to diseases peculiar to the tropics and developing countries for the same reasons.

We are grateful to Mr A. P. D. Wilcock for the preparation of specimens, Mr E. P. Daniels for photography, and Miss R. Bailey for redrawing some of the illustrations.

We must record our thanks for the employment in this and previous editions of photographs supplied by Professor N. P. L. Wildy, Professor D. McLean, Professor David Tyrrell, Dr R. W. Horne, Dr R. W. Riddell and Dr June Almeida and to Miss P. Leicester for three of the drawings.

Thanks are also due to the Controller, Her Majesty's Stationery Office for permission to include material in Figures 5.1, 7.4 and 8.1, to the publishers of the Proceedings of the Royal Society for Figure 2.3 and the American Review of Tuberculosis for Table 6.1.

London 1984   R.H.
                                                               E.M.C.

Contents

Micro-organisms, their discovery, structure and behaviour

Almost everyone is now aware that a great many diseases are caused by minute particles which have, over the years, been called by various names such as germs, microbes, bacteria, viruses and more recently, micro-organisms. They are all too small to be seen with the naked eye but are living things and therefore capable of reproducing themselves. They are, accordingly, sometimes present in enormous numbers in the tissues during the disease for which they are responsible. But although their existence had been suspected for many years, it was not until the invention of the compound optical micro-scope in 1835 that they were actually seen and described. Even so, this alone did not prove that they were the cause of the disease in which they were present, largely because very sim-ilar particles could also be found on the skin, in the throat and intestinal canal of perfectly normal people. Indeed, they were even known to be present in situations that have nothing to do with human beings or animals such as the atmosphere, soil, water and on vegetation.

   The fact that the organisms were actually the cause of the diseases in which they were found was eventually proved by the researches of the French scientist, Louis Pasteur and the German, Robert Koch. It was also shown that the micro-orga-nisms associated with disease were different in many respects from those found in normal persons or in inanimate Nature.

The first human infections shown to be due to particles of this nature were leprosy, puerperal fever, and boils, but by the end of the nineteenth century, the organisms responsible for many forms of wound infection and such diseases as tuberculosis, diphtheria, pneumonia, erysipelas, cerebro-spinal fever, tetanus, cholera, plague, dysentery and undulant fever were all identified.

Study of these organisms and proof that they were the cause of these diseases had been facilitated by the fact that they could be seen with the optical microscope and would grow in test tubes containing solutions of suitable foodstuffs. But towards the end of the nineteenth century it became clear that some diseases were almost certainly caused by living agents but which could not be seen or cultivated. This was first proved in the case of foot and mouth disease, an infection of cattle. Identification of similar agents responsible for diseases of human beings such as smallpox, poliomyelitis, yellow fever and influenza soon followed. Organisms of this description became known as viruses and following the invention of the electron microscope were shown to be extremely small particles.

While these advances were being made, a whole series of technical methods were evolved which facilitated the isolation and identification of micro-organisms of all kinds. This not only afforded considerable assistance in arriving at a correct diagnosis of illness but also led to detection of the sources of the organisms and the routes by which they had reached the patient. These discoveries had far reaching consequences because they led to the prevention of many of these diseases by measures that eliminated the sources of the organisms or prevented their reaching other persons. Such measures included sterilization by heat, filtration or antiseptics, the disposal and control of excreta and the eradication of insects. Because of this some post-operative infections, diseases carried by water such as typhoid fever and cholera and those conveyed by insects such as typhus and yellow fever became almost completely preventable.

A second development that started soon after the discovery of the part played by micro-organisms in the causation of disease was study of the mechanisms by which man and animals protect themselves against infection and recover from it after it has developed. Generally referred to as immunity, this has now become a science in itself much of which, nowadays, has little to do with micro-organisms. Nevertheless, one of its earliest but for all that, most important contributions was the discovery of the part played by antibodies in the prevention and cure of infection. These are new substances produced by the body cells as part of the reaction of the patient to the infection and which ultimately lead to destruction of the organisms or neutralization of the poisonous substances or toxins they produce. One of the consequences of this discovery was the demonstration of the value of vaccines, following whose administration, normal persons can be rendered immune to infection by certain organisms such as those responsible for diphtheria, smallpox, yellow fever, poliomyelitis and whooping cough.

The third development was the evolution of methods for the treatment of diseases caused by micro-organisms. The first for which this became possible was diphtheria which, it was found as early as 1891, could be cured by antibodies from a suitably immunized animal. The next advance came in 1910 when an arsenical compound was produced by the German worker, Paul Ehrlich, that could cure syphilis, yaws and relapsing fever. Another series of compounds the sulphonamides were also discovered by a German scientist, Gerhard Domagk, in 1935. These could cure such diseases as puerperal fever, erysipelas, gonorrhoea and one form of meningitis. But the most important advance of all was the discovery of the antibiotics. These are substances produced by moulds or bacteria. Penicillin, the most important, was discovered in 1928 by Sir Alexander Fleming but it was not until 1941 that its value was demonstrated by Sir Howard Florey and Sir Ernst Chain. Other antibiotics such as streptomycin, chloramphenicol and the tetracyclines soon followed. As a result of these discoveries, a great many diseases that were previously very severe and frequently led to death can now be cured quickly and easily.

This necessarily short account of the development of bacteriology and immunity illustrates the importance of both subjects in medical practice. For it is as a result of techniques based on them that so much disease can now be prevented and successfully treated. In all this, the nurse, wherever she may be, must play an active part. It is for this reason that she must know something about the micro-organisms that cause disease, their sources, the routes by which they travel and how the diseases they cause may be prevented and treated.

THE STRUCTURE OF MICRO-ORGANISMS

Although the micro-organisms dealt with in this book vary greatly in size and appearance, the great majority can be placed in one or other of three categories, viruses, bacteria and fungi. Each must be described in a little more detail.

The *viruses* are the smallest of the micro-organisms. Most of them cannot be seen even when using the highest powers of the optical microscope so that it is only with the aid of the electron microscope that any idea can be obtained of their size and shape. It is not necessary to describe all of them. Suffice it to say that the smallest, such as those responsible for poliomyelitis and yellow fever, are spherical with a diameter of only 0.00003 mm. The viruses that cause influenza are also spherical but considerably larger being about 0.0001 mm in diameter.

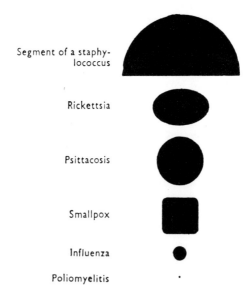

Segment of a staphylococcus

Rickettsia

Psittacosis

Smallpox

Influenza

Poliomyelitis

Fig. 1.1 Shapes and sizes of some of the smaller organisms. A segment of a staphylococcus is given for comparison.

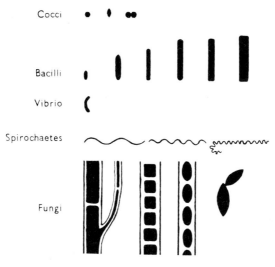

Fig. 1.2 The shapes and relative sizes of the bacteria and fungi.

Still larger are the viruses that cause smallpox and chickenpox which are cubes with sides about 0.0003 mm in length.

The chlamydiae and rickettsiae are sufficiently large to be visible with the optical microscope being spheres or ovals about 0.0003 mm in diameter. Although they resemble viruses in some ways, they are in fact, bacteria. They are responsible for typhus fever, trachoma and psittacosis.

The bacteria are all larger than these organisms and can therefore be readily seen with the optical microscope. Some are spheres, others are rods and still others are spirals.

The spherical organisms are usually referred to as *cocci*. They are about 0.001 mm in diameter. Some, such as the streptococci, are attached to each other in such a way that they form chains of anything from four to as many as twenty individual cocci. The remaining cocci do not form chains; but pneumococci, gonococci and meningococci may be attached to one another in pairs. The staphylococci, on the other hand, are usually arranged in cluster. Nothing is to be seen on the outer walls of any of these organisms except the pneumococcus; this possesses a semitransparent capsule.

The rods are known as *bacilli*. Their length and breadth vary considerably. One of the smallest, that responsible for undu-

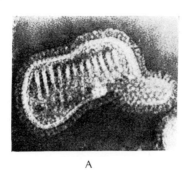 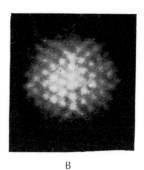

A   B

Fig. 1.3 (A), Electron microscope photograph of an influenza virus particle (Dr June Almeida). (B), Electron microscope photograph of an adenovirus particle (Dr R.W. Horne).

lant fever, resembles a slightly elongated coccus whereas the tubercle bacillus is a long thin rod. Most of them have nothing visible on their surfaces and assume no particular pattern in the microscope field. One of the exceptions is the anthrax bacillus which grows in the form of chains. Another is *Klebsiella* that forms capsules. Others possess *flagella* which are extremely thin hair-like processes attached to their outer walls. Some bacilli (those causing typhoid, paratyphoid and food infection) have large numbers along the sides of the rod whereas the cholera vibrio has a single flagellum attached at one end. Flagella are, undoubtedly, organs of locomotion which move backwards and forwards in the same way as the fins of a fish. Because of this, bacilli possessing them can be seen to move in a more or less deliberate manner when suspended in a watery fluid. There is, however, no evidence that ability to move in this way renders these organisms intrinsically more dangerous than those unable to do so.

It is usually impossible to distinguish any formed elements within the body of the bacillus without using special methods. But *spores* may be seen quite easily as completely transparent bodies cut off from the rest of the cell by a continuous coating. They are spherical, oval or oat shaped and can be formed at the centre of the bacillus or at one end. Many species produce them but of those responsible for human infections only those causing anthrax, gas gangrene, tetanus and botulism are able to do so.

Some of the bacilli are markedly curved and are called

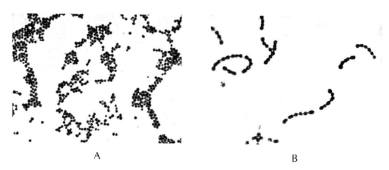

Fig. 1.4 (A) Staphylococci. (B) Streptococci.

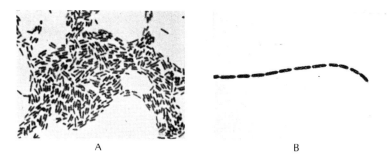

Fig. 1.5 (A) Coliform bacilli. (B)Anthrax bacilli.

vibrios. Because of their shape they are sometimes referred to as comma bacilli.

The spiral organisms or spirochaetes resemble corkscrews. The number of convolutions varies considerably; the spirochaete responsible for relapsing fever has only a few whereas that which causes leptospirosis or Weil's disease has so many that it may be very difficult to see the individual spirals. All the spirochaetes are actively motile.

The fungi are not only very much larger than the viruses and bacteria but are even more variable in size and appearance. The simplest is the organism responsible for thrush or moniliasis. It grows in the form of large slightly pointed cells. But most of the fungi form long filaments called *hyphae*. They are tubular with comparatively thick walls and with cross walls at intervals. They somewhat resemble bamboos. Square or oval bodies may develop within or on the sides of the hyphae whose importance will be discussed on page 14.

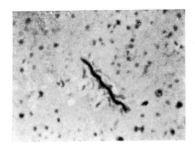

Fig. 1.6 Spirochaete of Vincent's angina.

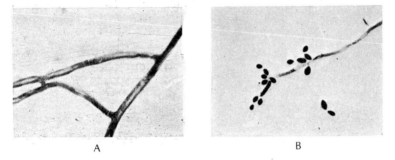

A   B

Fig. 1.7 A, Fungus of ringworm. B, *Candida albicans.*

MICRO-ORGANISMS AND THE PRODUCTION OF DISEASE

As already mentioned, micro-organisms are to be found every-where, in water, in soil, in the atmosphere, in vegetation, in food and drink, on our clothing and bedding and virtually everything else with which we come into contact. On the whole, the micro-organisms found in these situations are incapable of harming us by causing disease. On the contrary, many of them are of great value to us because it is due to their activities that dead bodies, dead vegetation and excreta are all decomposed and their chemical compounds rendered suitable for use by plants. In this way they play an important part in assuring our food supplies. But they also have much to do with the actual preparation of food and drink. The leavening of bread for example, is due to the formation of carbon dioxide as a result of the growth of the micro-organism that constitutes yeast. The fermentation of grape juice to produce wine is like-wise due to the growth of micro-organisms and is another example of the important part these minute forms of life can play in human affairs.

Another series of micro-organisms belonging to entirely different species are collectively known as *parasites* because they can only reproduce themselves under normal circumstances, in the tissues or on the surface of another form of life known as a *host* who provides them with food and shelter.

All living things act as hosts for some species of micro-organisms usually referred to as *commensals*. Indeed, not long after we are born, many species of organisms such as *Streptococcus viridans* and coliform bacilli get into our throats or intestinal canals where they remain as parasites for the rest of our lives. But they do not, except in unusual circumstances, cause disease; such organisms are called *commensals*.

As a general rule, they do us no harm and may even assist us in digesting our food. But in certain circumstances such as wasting diseases, malnutrition or exposure of the deep tissues as a result of injury, these organisms may produce infection usually referred to as *opportunistic infections*.

Other organisms usually called *pathogens* are not, as a rule, present in or on our persons until the early stages of an infection when they produce the symptoms characteristic of the disease because they are able to *invade* the tissues and form *toxins*. Invasion of the tissues produces the local signs of infection such as pain, oedema, erythema and the formation of pus with, in the more severe infections, invasion of the lymphatics or blood stream leading to widespread dissemination of the organisms. The toxins that are formed at the same time, produce many of the symptoms accompanying infection such as fever, increase in the pulse rate, headache, nausea and, in the more severe cases, delirium and death.

Nor are processes of this type confined to human beings for animals may suffer in much the same way. But in general, the micro-organisms responsible for disease in any one animal species are not likely to cause disease in any other species. Some organisms may, however, cause disease in more than one species. It is for this reason that such important human diseases as brucellosis and bubonic plague which are fundamentally diseases of cattle and rats respectively, may occur in human beings.

Organisms vary greatly in pathogenic activity but those

capable of causing severe infections with death as a possible ending, are usually referred to as *highly virulent*, whereas those that can only produce minor infections with quick recovery, possess only *low virulence*.

Diseases caused by micro-organisms

The viruses are responsible for many forms of infection. In some, such as smallpox, chickenpox, measles and german measles the virus particles get into the blood stream and so become widespread throughout the body. It is because of this that they can produce the rashes that are characteristic of these infections. Other viruses produce infections that are more localized. Those of influenza and the common cold, for example, generally confine their activities to the respiratory tract while the liver is the organ that is attacked in yellow fever, the skin in herpes simplex and the brain in encephalitis.

Another series of organisms are intermediate in size, and in some other characteristics between the viruses on the one hand and the bacteria on the other. These are the rickettsiae and chlamydiae, the former being responsible for the typhus fevers and the latter for trachoma, both diseases that are still common in underdeveloped countries.

The smallest of the bacteria are the cocci which tend to produce purulent infections, that is to say localized infections in which pus formation is a cardinal feature. The staphylococci cause this type of infection in the skin in the form of boils and carbuncles or in open wounds into which they have been able to penetrate. The streptococcus is responsible for infections of the throat such as tonsillitis and scarlet fever but it too may infect wounds. The gonococcus causes gonorrhoea, the meningococcus, meningitis, while the pneumococcus is a common cause of pneumonia.

One of the most important of the bacilli that are responsible for human infection is the tubercle bacillus. This can infect almost any organ, but the lung is by far the most usual. Almost as important are the bacilli that produce infections of the digestive tract such as food infection, dysentery, typhoid and paratyphoid fever. Open wounds may also be invaded by different bacilli such as *Pseudomonas, Proteus* and gas gangrene and tetanus bacilli. Other, much more unusual, infections caused by bacilli are brucellosis, anthrax, and diphtheria. The most important disease caused by vibrios is cholera, an extremely severe and frequently fatal infection of the intestinal tract.

The spirochaetes can be extremely formidable because the diseases they produce may be very severe and very disfiguring. Perhaps the worst is syphilis, but yaws, a disease of tropical countries, is very nearly as important. Relapsing fever, another spirochaetal infection, used to be common in Europe but is nowadays limited to Africa and is much less serious than syphilis or yaws. Leptospirosis is also due to spirochaetes. The organisms attack the liver to cause jaundice. Lastly, there is Vincent's angina, an ulcerative infection of the mouth.

The fungi are, on the whole, more important as causative agents of disease in tropical countries than in the temperate zones. In Great Britain, the commonest diseases caused by fungi are thrush, an infection of the mouth, ringworm in which the hair is attacked, and athlete's foot, a skin infection.

REPRODUCTION OF MICRO-ORGANISMS

Like all living things, micro-organisms must reproduce themselves in order to perpetuate the species. In general, this consists in division of the organisms into two identical halves. Under suitable conditions, this occurs as soon as the cell has grown to full size. A wall then begins to develop in the centre of the organism, along an equator if a coccus, and perpendicular to the long axis if a bacillus, vibrio or spirochaete. This wall soon becomes firm and continuous with the outer coating of the organism. In this way the organism literally cuts itself into two equal halves or daughter cells.

As a general rule, the two newly formed cells then separate. Smaller at first than the parent organism, they soon grow to full size and then reproduce themselves in exactly the same way. In the presence of abundant foodstuffs some organisms such as coliform bacilli may divide in this way every twenty or thirty minutes, but other organisms of which the tubercle bacillus is an example may require several days.

Viruses multiply in a very different manner. They cannot do so in lifeless artificial media. They require living cells. Once

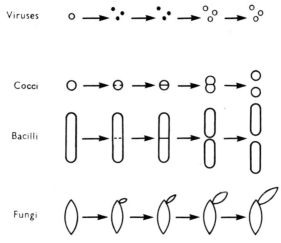

Fig. 1.8 Stages in the reproduction of the viruses, bacteria and fungi.

inside the cells, the nucleic acids in the virus particles then take control of the cell and direct its nucleus to produce new virus particles. This process upsets the economy of the invaded cell to such an extent that it dies and releases the newly formed virus particles into the surrounding tissues.

The fungi multiply in several different ways. That responsible for thrush is a relatively large oval which does not divide but forms *buds*. When reproduction occurs these buds are first seen as swellings on the surface not far from the ends and gradually enlarge until they are about the same size as the parent. At first they remain attached by their pointed ends but soon break loose and in due course may reproduce themselves in the same way. When the fungus forms a hypha as is the case with that which causes ringworm, the hypha may grow lengthways. As a result, a tangled mass of hyphae may be formed, sometimes referred to as a *mycelium*.

Spore formation and germination

When bacilli belong to species that are able to form spores, no spores are usually produced so long as the organisms are provided with adequate nourishment and are kept at a temperature suitable for reproduction. The bacilli multiply in exactly the same way as do those of non-sporing species.

Spore formation is, in a sense, a defensive measure on the part of the organism designed to perpetuate the species when the external conditions are such that the bacilli themselves could neither survive nor multiply. They accordingly tend to appear in the organisms when the food supply becomes deficient or the temperature is higher than usual. Once formed they can not only remain in a state of suspended animation more or less indefinitely, but they can survive treatment that would quickly kill the bacilli from which they were derived. They can, for example, resist strong antiseptics, drying, the action of sunlight and high temperatures. Some can even resist boiling water for as much as 15 minutes.

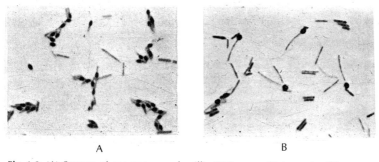

A   B

Fig. 1.9 (A) Spores of gas gangrene bacilli. (B) Spores of tetanus bacilli.

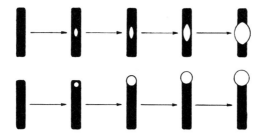

Fig. 1.10 The formation of spores.

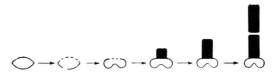

Fig. 1.11 Stages in the germination of a spore and the emergence of the vegetative form of the organism.

If, however, the spores are once again provided with food-stuffs and incubated at a suitable temperature, they then come to life again or *germinate*. The first step in this process is rupture of the coat and the second, the development of a young bacillus from within the spore. This soon grows to full size. Thenceforward it divides in the same way as do other bacilli and continues to do so until the factors once again operate that induce bacilli to form spores.

Fungi produce bodies such as arthrospores, chlamydospores and conidia which resembles bacterial spcres in many respects, particularly in their ability to remain alive for long pcriods and to produce hyphae when conditions are once again suitable for their germination.

CULTURE OF MICRO-ORGANISMS

When we suspect that micro-organisms are causing disease or we wish to ascertain that they have come from some external source such as food, water, dust, etc., microscopic examination of the material will not tell us whether pathogenic organisms are present. This may be due to the fact that there are too few organisms to be seen or that they are too small to be visible when using the ordinary optical microscope. But even if there are adequate numbers of organisms which are big enough to be seen with the microscope it is very often impossible to tell, by their appearance alone, whether they belong to a pathogenic or non-pathogenic species.

Identification becomes much easier, however if the micro-

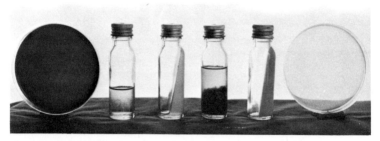

Fig. 1.12 Bacteriological media. Left to right: A blood agar plate, a tube of broth, an agar slope, Robertson's meat medium, Lowenstein medium for the growth of tubercle bacilli, an agar plate.

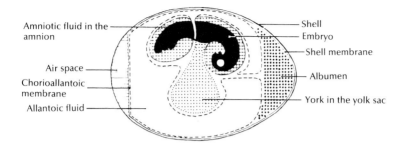

Fig. 1.13 Diagrammatic representation of the embryo and related structures of a hen's egg about the twelfth day of incubation.

organisms can be *cultivated*; that is, made to reproduce themselves away from the disease process. This not only enables us to see them more easily, but makes possible other methods of identification.

For cultivation the organisms must be provided with the conditions that imitate those that face them when they get into the human body. That is to say, they must be *incubated* at the same temperature as the human body, 37.5°C, and be provided with foodstuffs that resemble the proteins, carbohydrates, fats and vitamins they find in human tissues. Solutions containing them are usually referred to as *culture media*.

The simplest medium is *broth*. This can be made in many ways, but generally consists of a solution of the proteins, etc., present in meat. It is in fact a thin soup closely resembling consommé. For many organisms it may be necessary to enrich it by the addition of certain vitamins, carbohydrates or blood. Many species of organisms grow readily in a liquid medium of this description forming a more or less opaque cloud. In time, the organisms constituting this cloud settle to the bottom of the tube in the form of a mass.

For many purposes it is desirable to use a *solid medium*. This may be made in a number of ways but by far the most useful consists of broth containing a gelatinous substance extracted from seaweed known as agar. The mixture is liquid when hot but when allowed to cool it solidifies. If the medium has been put into a test tube, a smooth sheet of medium with a firm surface can be obtained. It is usually referred to as an *agar slope*. It is more usual for the medium to be allowed to set in a flat glass container called a *petri dish*. Bacteria or fungi smeared over the surface of such a solid medium and incubated at body temperature, will multiply rapidly. In the process, they form *colonies* which consist of piled up masses of organisms on the surface of the medium.

Although media made in this way suffice for the growth of practically all the bacteria and fungi, they are completely valueless for the cultivation of the viruses. These organisms have become so highly specialized that they do not produce all the enzymes required to digest the proteins, carbohydrates and fats in culture media. The only way by which they can reproduce themselves is by invading a living cell and ultilizing the enzymes of the cell. In a sense they borrow the digestive apparatus of their host to enable them to grow and reproduce themselves. Indeed they go even further, for the cell provides the foodstuffs as well.

For the *cultivation of viruses*, special methods are therefore necessary, all of which provide living cells in one form or another. Perhaps the simplest is to use the living cells in a *laboratory animal*. The virus is injected into the tissues known to be most suitable for its growth. After a suitable interval, the animal is killed. The tissues are then ground up with sand and saline. The virus particles in the cells are, in this way, released into the saline. For many years this was the only method by which suspensions of viruses could be obtained for study.

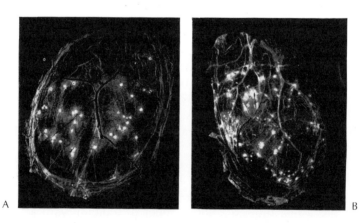

Fig. 1.14 Growth of viruses in the chorioallantoic membrane of the developing egg. (A) Herpes simplex (Dr N.L.P. Wildy). (B) Murray Valley encephalitis (Dr D.M. McLean).

Needless to say such methods are crude and expensive and in the course of the years, others have been evolved. One of the most useful is to employ *fertile eggs* of the domestic fowl. When such eggs are incubated at 35–37°C, the embryo starts to develop and grows so rapidly that 21 days later the fully grown chick emerges from the shell. During the intermediate phases of its development, however, it can be employed for the growth of many viruses. All that is required is to inject the suspension of virus into the embryo or its attached membranes and incubate the egg for two or more days longer. The virus multiplies in the cells and heavy suspensions of the virus may be obtained from the fluids or tissues of the embryo.

More recently it has been found possible to employ *tissue cultures*. These consist of living cells derived from such sources as the kidneys of monkeys, the embryos of chickens, or the human amnion. These are suspended in solutions containing all the salts, vitamins, etc., necessary for the survival and growth of the cells.

The cells remain alive and may even divide to produce sheets of new cells on the walls of the container. If to such preparations virus particles are added, they invade the cells multiply inside them and then escape into the fluid. Methods of this description are extensively used nowadays not only for the diagnosis of virus infection but for the large-scale production of poliomyelitis vaccine.

DIFFERENTIATION OF MICRO-ORGANISMS

The tests evolved for this purpose are legion and it is quite unnecessary for medical students, and still less for nurses, to have more than a general idea as to how micro-organisms are differentiated from one another. This generally involves study of their appearance under the microscope, their staining reactions, the type of colony produced when grown on a solid medium and their behaviour in biochemical and serological tests. These must be discussed in more detail.

Microscopic appearance

Because of their size, an electron microscope is essential for

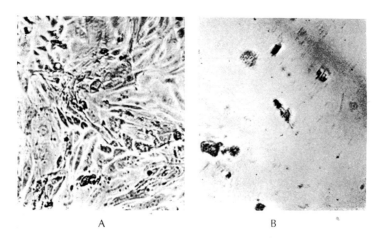

A   B

Fig. 1.15 Growth of a virus in tissue culture. (A) normal intact cells before addition of the virus. (B) cells completely disrupted as a result of growth of poliomyelitis virus.

the very small organisms such as the viruses. They must first be dried in a very thin film which is then *shadowed*. As a result of this the virus particles appear under the microscope as though they were standing up in bright sunlight with deep shadows cast to one side. By this method, it is possible to obtain so good an idea of their size, shape and surface configuration that this procedure has been successfully employed for the diagnosis of smallpox.

The larger organisms such as the cocci and bacilli can be seen quite easily with the optical microscope. For this purpose they are dried on a microscope slide and then *stained*. This enables us to determine their shape, size and whether or not they possess surface structures such as capsules or flagella. Information obtained in this way can be of considerable assistance.

Staining reactions

When organisms have been stained it is usually possible to remove the colouring matter from the organisms with solvents such as strong acids, alcohol or acetone. But if the organisms contain certain chemical compounds these may form so strong a union with some of the dyes that the organisms do not become decolourized. This is an easy method for detecting the presence of such substances. The method of differentiation known as *Gram's stain* depends on this principle. By its aid it is possible to show that organisms such as staphylococci and gonococci which appear alike when examined under the microscope belong to different species. For staphylococci retain the stain and are *Gram positive* whereas gonococci do not and are, accordingly, *Gram negative*.

A second substance that can modify the staining reactions of bacteria is a waxy material incorporated in the walls of the organisms. This is detected in the Ziehl Neelsen method of staining in which once a stain has penetrated the wax and reached the interior of the organism it cannot be removed by the application of strong acid or alcohol. Such organisms are said to be *acid fast*. The tubercle bacillus, the leprosy bacillus and certain related species belong to this category.

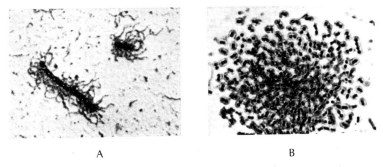

A   B

Fig. 1.16 (A) Flagella of *Proteus vulgaris*. (B) Capsules of pneumococci.

Appearance of the colonies

A second and very important method of differentiation is the shape, size, colour and consistency of the colonies produced on solid media. This is due to the fact that each species generally produces such distinctive colonies that a skilled observer may be able to tell at a glance what variety of organisms have formed the colony. Further useful information may also be obtained if blood, certain sugars or chemical compounds be present in the medium because they may be acted upon by some species but not by others.

Biochemical tests

During multiplication, micro-organisms can act upon many different chemical compounds, but in general those acted upon by one species are not the same as those attacked by other, even closely related species. Employing media containing the substances found most useful for the differentiation of the particular species being studied, it may be possible by this method to name the organism at once by ascertaining whether or not the substance has been acted upon.

The actual compounds employed are much too numerous and the details of the tests themselves too technical to warrant further description of these methods, but some such tests are nearly always necessary to confirm the provisional diagnosis based on the appearance of the organism and its colonies.

Serological reactions

Study of micro-organisms by chemical methods has shown that they all contain proteins and carbohydrates, but that those formed by one species are specific for that species. That is to say, their chemical constitution is different from the compounds formed by every other species of micro-organisms. Using the methods of the chemical laboratory it would, theoretically, be possible to name any micro-organism by analyses of its constituent proteins and carbohydrates. This would be a formidable undertaking but fortunately the same information can be obtained by serological methods which are very much simpler.

These depend upon the fact that if a suspension of killed micro-organisms be injected a number of times into an animal such as a rabbit, the animal reacts by producing *antibodies*. These are released into the blood and are present in the serum after the blood has clotted.

The antibodies formed in this way will only react with the chemical substances of the particular species of micro-organisms injected into the animal. Thus the serum of the animal can be employed as a reagent for the detection of this particular species of micro-organism.

Several methods may be employed for the actual tests, but that which is generally used is the *agglutination reaction*. This depends upon the fact that if an antibody capable of reacting with the organism is present in the serum it combines with the organisms which then adhere to one another and form clumps that are visible to the naked eye. Other species of organisms mixed with the serum will remain discrete and unagglutinated.

Other methods such as the *fluorescent antibody technique* and the *precipitin* and *complement fixation reactions* do not need description but they are all fundamentally the same as the agglutination reaction in that they detect combination between the antibody and the chemical substances produced by the organisms.

NOMENCLATURE OF MICRO-ORGANISMS

As a result of these procedures it is almost always possible to isolate and identify any micro-organism whatever its origin. It can then be named. Bacteriologists use for this purpose the Linnaean system of nomenclature in which the first name denotes the Genus and the second the Species. Thus, the organism responsible for boils belongs to a genus called *Staphylococcus*. This genus also contains another variety of organism which not only does not cause boils but is dissimilar in other respects as well. It is, therefore, a member of a different species. Largely because it forms milky white colonies, it is called *Staphylococcus albus* while that which causes boils is called *Staphylococcus aureus* because its colonies are golden yellow in colour.

Use of this system presupposes a knowledge of Latin. But for practical purposes it is not really necessary and will not, therefore, be employed in this book. Instead, a much simpler system will be employed in which, as far as possible the organism will be known by the name of the disease for which it is responsible. Thus, *Mycobacterium tuberculosis*, the correct name for the organism that causes tuberculosis, will be referred to as 'the tubercle bacillus'; *Salmonella typhi* as 'the typhoid bacillus' and so on.

Unfortunately, it is not possible to employ this system for all organisms largely because some are not associated with any particular disease. To employ the Linnaean names would require memorization of two words and there may even be several species that behave in the same way. But since the Generic name usually serves, this alone will be employed. For this reason, *Pseudomonas aeruginosa*, used in previous editions, now becomes *Pseudomonas*, and *Proteus vulgaris* simply *Proteus*. Several other organisms whose nomenclature has also become unsatisfactory will be re-named. *Haemophilus influenzae* previously referred to as 'the influenza bacillus' has no connection with true influenza for which reason it will be called *Haemophilus*. Similarly, 'Friedländers bacillus' becomes *Klebsiella*. A third is the organism responsible for thrush, hitherto referred to as 'the fungus of thrush'. Since it may cause other very different types of infection, it is better called *Candida*.

Once it is known that an infection is due to a certain variety of organism, it becomes possible to initiate treatment with the correct antibiotic or other drug and to attempt to ascertain the source of the organism so that further cases may be prevented. For these reasons identification of the organisms causing disease may be a matter of considerable practical importance.

2

Infection and immunity

Before it is possible to prevent or cure infections by micro-organisms, it is necessary to have some idea of the diseases involved, the manner in which the illness develops and the processes by which the patient combats the organisms. It is with such matters that this chapter is concerned.

THE PRODUCTION OF DISEASE BY MICRO-ORGANISMS

It is extremely probable that when we become infected by micro-organisms, the number of bacterial cells that start the process by getting into our tissues is very small indeed. If, moreover, they do not multiply, they will produce no symptoms, even though they may succeed in remaining alive. But if multiplication does occur, the invasion of the tissues and the production of toxins are the cause of the symptoms.

Although this is, fundamentally, the mode of causation of all diseases due to micro-organisms, there are two and possibly more exceptions in which the organisms themselves need not enter our bodies at all for they attack us by producing toxins as a result of their multiplication in certain types of food before it is eaten. But not very long after it has been swallowed, the toxins and not the organisms themselves, begin to cause symptoms.

One of the organisms that can do this is the bacillus responsible for botulism—a fatal but fortunately very rare disease—described in more detail on page 189. The second is the staphylococcus, certain strains of which can multiply in foods containing milk or cream, such as trifles, custards or cakes, and produce a toxin that causes acute diarrhoea and vomiting soon after the food is eaten. This is particularly liable to occur in hot weather and many weddings and similar festivities have been marred by large numbers of the guests being taken ill in this way.

With these exceptions, it is the multiplication of the organisms in the tissues that causes the signs and symptoms of disease. But it is obvious that this can only occur if the organisms are able to get into our bodies. At first sight, there should be no difficulty about this for they are to be found in large numbers in our environment. They are certainly present in enormous numbers in water, soil, excreta, manure, sewage, the decomposing bodies of animals and rotting vegetation. Smaller but still large numbers are to be found in the air and in our food, tap water and milk. Our clothing too is heavily contaminated, as are our homes, with large numbers on the furniture, curtains, bedding, floors and walls. Nor do these organisms lack opportunity to cause infection for some enter our bodies with every inspiration we take and every meal we eat, and every time we cut or scratch ourselves they can reach the deeper layers of the skin and sometimes the subcutaneous tissues as well.

Nevertheless, despite the abundant supply of micro-organisms and their many opportunities of reaching various parts of our anatomy, these encounters are only seldom followed by the signs and symptoms indicative of active infection. The reasons for this comparative freedom from infection will be discussed later, but even when an organism is capable of producing disease the number of patients it infects and the manner in which it behaves in the community generally vary considerably.

Some pathogenic organisms do not exist at all in certain parts of the world. The virus of measles, for example, may be absent for long periods from such remote places as Greenland

and northern Canada largely because patients in the acute stage of the disease do not get there and so provide the virus necessary to produce further cases of the disease.

A second reason for the absence of organisms is that the vehicles that transport them from person to person and so keep them alive in the community, may themselves be absent. In consequence, the organisms die out, even if they succeed in reaching the community in question. This particularly applies to diseases that require insects for their transmission. Yellow fever is one such disease. The virus that causes it can only pass from person to person if it is transported by a certain variety of mosquito. But this mosquito is unable to breed in a cold climate and it is for this reason that the disease it carries has always confined itself to hot countries such as those of Central America, the Caribbean and Central Africa.

A third and increasingly important reason for the absence of organisms is that thanks to various measures, Man himself can eradicate or control these organisms so successfully that the diseases they produce likewise disappear or become very rare. This particularly applies to those responsible for intestinal infections such as cholera, typhoid and paratyphoid fevers which can be almost completely eradicated by sanitation. They have, therefore, become very uncommon indeed in countries with good sanitation but still occur in developing countries such as Egypt, India and China.

But even when the organisms in question are present at all times and in adequate numbers the number of patients infected may vary considerably from time to time. It is, for example, well known that infections of the respiratory tract such as pneumonia, colds and influenza are more likely to occur in winter than in summer, whereas poliomyelitis and some of the intestinal infections are much commoner in the late summer than in the winter months.

Thus, many factors may play a part in determining what infections are likely to occur, when they will occur and how often. But in general micro-organisms attack human beings in four different ways:

1. Some organisms usually produce what are known as *sporadic infections* in which they infect one person in a town or village while the rest of the inhabitants go scot free. The next patient to be infected, sometimes long afterwards and

living miles away, may have had no contact whatever with the first patient. The organisms responsible for undulant fever, leptospirosis, puerperal fever and tetanus generally behave in this way.

2. Another series of organisms, notably, *Proteus, Pseudomonas, Bacteroides* and *Candida*, seldom attack those in good health but may do so if the normal immunity has fallen as a result of the use of cytotoxic drugs or if the local conditions in the tissues are unusually favourable for the development of infection. These are frequently referred to as *opportunistic infections*.

3. The great majority of pathogenic organisms, particularly those responsible for chickenpox, mumps, common colds, scarlet fever, tuberculosis, pneumonia and wound infections, produce *endemic infections*. In these, the number of patients infected varies little from year to year.

4. Micro-organisms may also produce *epidemics*. These are outbreaks of disease in which large numbers of people are attacked within a few days, following which the epidemic disappears. Influenza, cholera, and smallpox are almost always epidemic diseases. Although many epidemics are limited to a town or village, whole countries may be involved. Indeed, influenza may attack almost all countries in the world to produce what is frequently called a *pandemic*.

DISEASES CAUSED BY MICRO-ORGANISMS

It is not within the scope of this book to describe each of the diseases that may be caused by micro-organisms but it may assist students if they know which of the many forms of disease likely to afflict human beings are caused by them, the organs in the body that will probably be attacked and the particular variety of organism usually responsible. This is given in the form of a summary in Table 2.1. Further information about these diseases and the organisms themselves will be found in Chapters 10–15.

Table 2.1 Diseases caused by micro-organisms

Principal site of infection	Micro-organism responsible
Generalized infections	
Smallpox (Variola)	Smallpox virus
Chickenpox (Varicella)	Chickenpox virus
Measles	Measles virus
Rubella (German measles)	Rubella virus
Typhoid and Paratyphoid fevers (Enteric)	Typhoid and paratyphoid bacilli
Relapsing fever	Relapsing fever spirochaete
Typhus fever	Typhus rickettsia
Plague	Plague bacillus
Brucellosis (Undulant fever)	Brucellosis bacillus
Dengue	Dengue virus
Bornholm disease	Coxsackie virus
Nose and throat	
Common cold	Common cold virus
Influenza	Influenza virus
Tonsillitis and scarlet fever	Haemolytic streptococcus
Diphtheria	Diphtheria bacillus
Mouth	
Vincent's angina	Vincent's angina spirochaete
Thrush	*Candida*
Actinomycosis	*Actinomyces*
Mumps	Mumps virus
Trachea, bronchi and lungs	
Bronchitis	*Haemophilus*
Lobar pneumonia	Pneumococcus
Virus pneumonia (Primary atypical pneumonia)	*Mycoplasma*
Whooping cough	Whooping cough bacillus
Tuberculosis	Tubercle bacillus
Q fever	Q fever rickettsia
Intestinal canal	
Food infection (Food poisoning)	Salmonella
Infantile gastro-enteritis	Coliform bacillus
Enterotoxic poisoning	Staphylococcus. Gas gangrene bacillus
Dysentery	Dysentery bacilli
Cholera	Cholera vibrio
Urinary tract	
Pyelitis and cystitis	Coliform bacillus, *Proteus*
Tuberculosis	Tubercle bacillus

Table 2.1 (continued)

Genital tract	
Syphilis	Syphilis spirochaete
Gonorrhoea	Gonococcus
Lymphogranuloma inguinale	Lymphogranuloma organism
Non-specific urethritis	*Mycoplasma*
Puerperal fever	Haemolytic streptococcus
	Anaerobic streptococcus
Liver	
Infective hepatitis	Infective hepatitis virus
Serum hepatitis (Homologous serum jaundice)	Serum hepatitis virus
Leptospirosis	Leptospirosis spirochaete
Yellow fever	Yellow fever virus
Central nervous system	
Meningitis	Menningococcus, *Haemophilus,* Pneumococcus, Tubercle bacillus
Encephalitis	Encephalitis virus
Poliomyelitis	Poliomyelitis virus
Rabies	Rabies virus
Botulism	Botulism bacillus
Eyes	
Conjunctivitis	Pneumococcus, Staphylococcus, *Haemophilus*, Adenoviruses
Trachoma, Inclusion blepharitis	Trachoma organism
Skin	
Furunculosis, Boils, Carbuncles, Impetigo, Paronychia	Staphylococcus
Ringworm, Tinea pedis	Ringworm fungi
Erysipelas	Haemolytic streptococcus, Staphylococcus
Herpes	Herpes virus
Herpes zoster (Shingles)	Herpes zoster virus
Leprosy	Leprosy bacillus
Yaws	Yaws spirochaete
Pinta	Pinta spirochaete
Anthrax	Anthrax bacillus
Wounds, burns and scalds	
Pyogenic infection	Staphylococcus, Haemolytic streptococcus, *Pseudomonas, Proteus,*
Gas gangrene	Gas gangrene bacillus
Tetanus	Tetanus bacillus

THE REACTION OF HUMAN BEINGS TO MICRO-ORGANISMS

Although we live in a world abundantly supplied with micro-organisms, we do not become infected very often. This is partly due to the fact that the great majority of these organisms are quite incapable of survival and multiplication in the proteins of which our bodies are constructed and at the comparatively high temperatures at which they are maintained. Indeed, to many species of micro-organisms, the human body is about as inhospitable as is a desert island to us.

Nevertheless, a great many of the remaining species of organisms can utilize our proteins as foodstuffs for, after death, all the soft parts are decomposed by their activities within a few months leaving only the more indigestible skeleton intact. It is obvious therefore that so long as we are alive, we evidently possess protective mechanisms that enable us to keep our bodies free from the attentions of many species of micro-organisms.

These protective mechanisms can, however, be breached for at longer or shorter intervals we suffer from some form of infection, with organisms multiplying in our tissues and producing symptoms of varying degrees of severity. More often than not, we recover without permanent injury of any kind. Here too we must evidently possess mechanisms that enable us to overcome attack by micro-organisms that have broken through the defences.

The mechanisms that enable us to escape the attention of organisms in general and to overcome those that do cause infection are two important aspects of the science of *immunity* and form the subject of the remainder of this chapter.

The mechanisms of defence

All living things have evolved methods by which they can protect themselves against the micro-organisms in their environnent. Some operate on the body surfaces and the mucous membranes, while others come into play when the deeper tissues are in danger.

Surface defences

Skin. So long as it is intact, the skin acts as a mechanical barrier which prevents organisms reaching the tissues beneath. But in addition to this it can also kill many varieties of organisms which reach it. In consequence such organisms as the typhoid bacillus may quickly disappear soon after getting on to the skin.

Mucous membranes. Like the skin, the mucous membranes also act as a mechanical barrier preventing access of organisms to the tissues below. But they can also kill micro-organisms that reach their surfaces. The tears, nasal mucus and saliva, for example, all contain an enzyme known as lysozyme which can rapidly kill most of the organisms that reach these surfaces from the air.

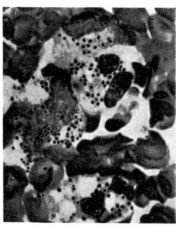

Fig. 2.1 Phagocytosis of micro-organisms by the white cells in human blood.

Inner defences

Whenever organisms reach the tissues beneath the skin or mucous membrane, they encounter two very important anti-bacterial mechanisms known as *phagocytosis* and *bacteriolysis*.

Phagocytosis. Many years ago, the Russian bacteriologist Metchnikoff showed that in all parts of the body, there are comparatively large cells which can engulf any solid particle that comes into contact with them. Micro-organisms come within this category and are similarly taken up. To do this, the

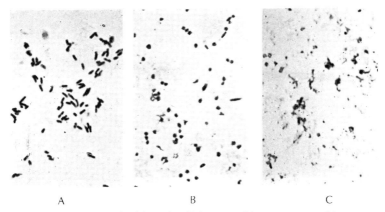

A   B   C

Fig. 2.2 Bacteriolysis of coliform bacilli by normal human serum. (A) immediately after mixing; (B) after 15 minutes; (C) after 30 minutes.

cell thrusts a finger-like projection of protoplasm towards the organism, surrounding it in such a way that when the projection is withdrawn into the body of the cell, the organism goes with it. Enzymes within the cell usually act upon the organism so that it is killed and may even be digested within a few minutes of its having been taken up by the cell.

Destruction of micro-organisms reaching the tissues begins within a few minutes of their arrival and even if some of them escape and are carried in the lymph stream to the nearest lymphatic gland, they can be dealt with equally expeditiously by similar phagocytic cells in the gland. If the organisms reach the venules and so get into the blood stream another set of cells in the liver and lungs can deal with them in the same way.

Bacteriolysis. In addition to phagocytosis, some species of organism can be rendered harmless by an entirely different mechanism known as bacteriolysis. This is due to the presence in the body fluids of two substances, properdin, and complement, which can so weaken the outer wall of the organism that water can get into it. This causes swelling and ultimately, bursting of the organism, leaving nothing more than a little formless debris.

Colonization of the tissues

Although the mechanisms described above the extraordinarily efficient and keep our bodies free from the attentions of the vast majority of the micro-organisms that reach them every day, some are endowed with properties that enable them to survive and multiply in or on the body surfaces. This need not invariably result in clinical infection. Such is the case with organisms that are usually referred to as *Commensals*. Being able to survive and multiply in the hair follicles and sweat glands of the skin or on the surface of the mucous membranes of the nose, throat and intestinal canal, they are acquired soon after birth and remain permanent inhabitants of these areas throughout the life of the host. It is only under somewhat unusual circumstances such as wasting diseases, avitaminosis and certain diseases of the blood, that such organisms are likely to produce active infections. It is usually under such circumstances that the so-called *opportunistic infections* are produced.

Another series of organisms known collectively as *pathogens* are much less likely to be present in or on our bodies without producing disease. They are usually acquired from another human being by processes described in more detail in the following chapter. Their ability to produce disease would seem to depend on their possessing certain chemical compounds on their surfaces that act as a protective armour and so enable them to resist both the outer and inner defensive mechanisms of the body. The substances in question are extremely elaborate carbohydrates or proteins which form either a capsule surrounding the organism or an envelope on its outer wall.

But even if the organism which has established itself in the tissues is a pathogen, it never produces the signs and symptoms of infection at once. For there is invariably an interval known as the *incubation period* between its arrival and the start of the symptoms.

Incubation period. In many infections, such as colds, scarlet fever and diphtheria only about 48 hours or so elapse before the organisms are sufficiently numerous to cause symptoms, but in others, the incubation period is very much longer. In typhoid fever, smallpox and measles, for example, it is 10 to 14 days, in infective hepatitis three weeks and in serum hepatitis it may be as long as three months. It is still a matter for conjecture as to why so long an incubation period should be necessary, but from animal experiments it would seem probable that during it the organisms may become widely disseminated in the body, but without causing any symptoms whatsoever.

Development of the infection

Once the incubation period is over, the organisms can then begin to produce the signs and symptoms associated with the disease for which they are responsible. To do this, it is necessary for the organisms to do two things—invade the tissues and form poisons or toxins.

Invasion of the tissues. To produce the signs and symptoms of infection the organisms must be able to spread through the tissues and in the process produce injury to neighbouring cells and other structures. To facilitate this some organisms produce certain substances called *spreading factors* that digest some of the compounds in the surrounding tissues. As a general rule, this local dissemination is eventually brought to a halt, the symptoms abate and the injured area is repaired. Unfortunately, some organisms are not content with so limited a field of activity and show marked tendencies to travel along the lymphatics to the lymphatic glands or into the veins to reach the blood stream. As a result, widespread injury to the local tissues and to important organs such as the lungs, heart and brain may be produced. Death too is more likely to occur than when the organisms remain localized.

Under most circumstances, the invasion of the blood stream can best be described as a leakage of comparatively small numbers of organisms into the circulation. But very rarely, there may be a sudden flooding of the blood stream by large numbers to produce profound shock that may lead to death within 24 hours. This is known as *septic* or *bacteraemic shock.*

Production of toxins. Accompanying all forms of infection, there are general symptoms such as headache, nausea, vomiting and delirium which become progressively worse if the disease is likely to end in death. In the great majority of infections these symptoms are probably due to *endotoxins* liberated from the organisms as a result of their dissolution in the tissues by enzymes. They are poisonous substances which probably owe much of their activity to their ability to produce changes in the blood vessels resembling those seen in secondary shock.

A few species produce another series of poisons called *exotoxins* which are not only very much more powerful but have more circumscribed activities. That formed by tetanus bacilli for example acts on the nervous system to produce exactly the same symptoms as those of the disease itself. That produced by the bacillus of botulism brings about the same paralyses of the cranial nerves as seen in the disease. That formed by the diphtheria bacillus produces degeneraton of the myocardium and the palsies of the throat, palate and eyes also seen in the more severe cases of diphtheria.

Death from infection

It is still not clear why some patients die as a result of infection when others, infected by the same species of organism, recover. But it would seem that some die because they have had the ill luck to be infected by certain strains of the organism which possess unusual abilities to invade the tissues and produce toxins. Others die for an entirely different reason— because their immunity apparatus cannot respond soon enough or adequately enough to enable them to over-come the invading organisms and neutralize the poisons they produce.

Recovery from infection

In the great majority of infections recovery occurs and the organisms disappear at the onset of convalescence. It might, therefore, be thought that recovery is merely due to inability of the organisms to go on multiplying and so remain alive in the patient. This, however, is most improbable, for in some infections such as scarlet fever, diphtheria and typhoid fever the organisms may not only persist in the throat or intestinal canal of some of the patients for many months after they have completely recovered, but remain fully virulent and capable of causing infection if they reach a susceptible individual. This suggests that recovery is not due to inability of the organisms to go on multiplying but that it is because some change has occurred in the patient as a result of which the organisms are prevented from causing further local damage and their toxins are rendered harmless.

Thus whatever has altered as a result of the infection it is not the organism but the patient. Confirmation of this is afforded by the very old observation that once we have recovered from many forms of infection of which measles, chickenpox, diphtheria and mumps are good examples, we are no longer susceptible to these diseases so that we are not likely to suffer a second attack no matter how long we live.

A great deal of study has been devoted to ascertaining what are the alterations in the tissues that enable us to bring an infection to a halt and enable us to resist further attacks by the same organism for the rest of our lives. There seems to be little doubt that both are fundamentally due to the same mechanism; the acquisition of new powers by the patient which enable him to kill the pathogenic organism concerned more easily and quickly than is possible for normal persons and to neutralize the toxins they form before they reach vital centres such as the brain or heart.

A patient who has acquired new powers of this description is said to possess *immunity* to the organism concerned. The processes that bring this about are obviously of importance and require further comment.

IMMUNITY TO MICRO-ORGANISMS

Until quite recently it was generally assumed that ability to protect ourselves against infection and recovery from it depended on the formation and presence in the fluid portion of the circulating blood of new substances called *antibodies*. In this process certain specialized cells also play a secondary but nonetheless important part. But in some infections, it is now known that it is cells rather than antibodies that play the predominant role. For this reason it is necessary to have some idea of the cells involved before it is possible to discuss immunity as a whole.

Cells connected with immunity

For the development of both types of immune response *lymphocytes* are of considerable importance. They are small cells and their nuclei take up most of the cell. Some are known as

B lymphocytes and are named after the Bursa of Fabricius an organ found in chickens but not in Man. Human B lymphocytes come from the lymphoid tissue associated with the gut. When suitably stimulated the B lymphocytes become the *plasma cells* that produce the antibodies that play so important a part in immunity.

The T lymphocytes, on the other hand, are so called because they are associated with the thymus gland. They produce soluble substances which activate *macrophages* so that they can kill micro-organisms. Macrophages are large motile cells and can crawl along surfaces towards the organisms which they phagocyte and destroy. They are found circulating in the blood and are also fixed in the tissues and they play a very important part in clearing the blood stream of bacteria. Somewhat smaller are the *polymorphonuclear cells*,.so called because their nuclei consist of what appears to be a thin thread of nuclear material with from one to three or even more swellings. These cells are also motile and can phagocyte and destroy micro-organisms. They are in fact the main constituent of the pus produced in many forms of infection.

Types of immunity

In view of the fact that the micro-organisms that may infect human beings range in size from the minute mass of the nucleoprotein constituting the virus that causes poliomyelitis to the relatively enormous bacillus responsible for anthrax and the even larger and still more complicated fungus that causes ringworm, it is perhaps not surprising that the mechanisms that enable us to protect ourselves against and recover from infections are not all the same. And certainly two very different mechanisms are now known. Some are dealt with by what is known as *cell mediated immunity* whereas others are combated by a very different process not so far given a name but which for the sake of convenience can be called *antibody mediated immunity*. Both must be discussed in some detail.

Antibody mediated immunity

In the great majority of infections the principal factor involved in immunity would seem to be the formation by the plasma cells of one or more antibodies that become part of the fluid portion of the circulating blood and are thereby carried to the infected area. They are a specialized type of protein consisting of globulin and are not as a rule present before the infection but make their appearance about the time of recovery and frequently persist in the plasma for long periods afterwards, sometimes for many years.

Antibodies facilitate recovery from infection and protect against further infection in a number of ways all of which depend on their ability to combine with compounds present in or on the organisms or with the soluble substances they produce such as the toxins. Because of this some antibodies render inert the substances on the surface of the organisms that protect them against destruction by phagocytosis or by bacteriolysis. Another series of antibodies render the toxins and other poisonous products innocuous. Antibodies also play an important part in protection against infection by viruses in

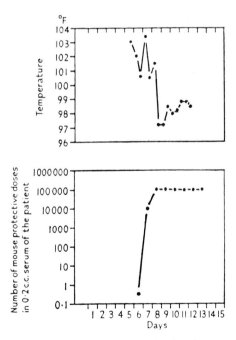

Fig. 2.3 Development of mouse protective antibodies for pneumococci during pneumonia (data from R. R. Armstrong, 1925, *Proc. Roy. Soc.*, B**98**, 525).

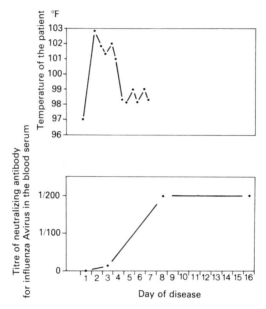

Fig. 2.4 Appearance of neutralizing antibody for influenza virus in the course of an attack of influenza.

that they combine with the virus particles in such a manner that they are unable to enter the cells in which they must multiply if they are to cause active infection. Thus the organisms in a sense encompass their own destruction for the antibodies, once formed, eventually reach the infected area and bring about death of the organisms and neutralization of their toxic products.

The cells that produce antibodies are stimulated to do so by chemical compounds collectively known as *antigens*. Consisting of proteins or compounds of protein and carbohydrate, some such as the toxins are already in solution when they leave the organisms. Others form part of the body of the organisms but go into solution when, as invariably happens some of organisms in the infected area undergo dissolution. Once in solution, they are carried to the antibody producing cells by way of the circulating blood.

Although the sources from which these compounds come disappear when the infection is over, antibodies continue to be produced probably because the cells have been 'educated' to do so even when the antigen is no longer available. Nevertheless, the antibody level of the blood does not rise because antibodies once formed, tend to disappear at about the same rate as new antibody is produced. In consequence, the antibodies may be found in the circulating blood for months and even years following the infection and it is for this reason that second attacks of such infections as measles, diphtheria, scarlet fever and smallpox are so unusual.

Specificity of antibodies

Although antibodies play an important part in combating many organisms, it is a matter of some importance that they will only combine with and so render innocuous the particular chemical compounds (antigens) that stimulated their production. But those produced by staphylococci, for example, are chemically different from those produced by typhoid bacilli or, in fact, any other organism. In consequence, the antibodies that assisted a patient to combat a staphylococcal infection are valueless for typhoid fever or any other infection.

Production of antibodies in the absence of clinical infection

In view of the fact that it is chemical substances from the organisms that stimulate the plasma cells to produce antibodies, it is perhaps not surprising that they may also be produced when there is no sign of clinical infection. This can be brought about in several different ways.

Subclinical infection. It is not unusual for a pathogenic organism to reach the tissues where it may survive and multiply but without producing all the signs and symptoms of the disease, going no further than causing a transitory and indefinite illness or possibly no symptoms at all. But in spite of the benign nature of this form of infection, it is quite sufficient to stimulate the antibody-forming cells to produce the antibodies that are necessary to combat the organisms if, some time later, the individual encounters them again. The organisms responsible for many infections such as diphtheria, scarlet fever, mumps, whooping cough and poliomyelitis may behave in this way and it is for this reason that many of us are known to possess antibodies for the organisms concerned in spite of the fact

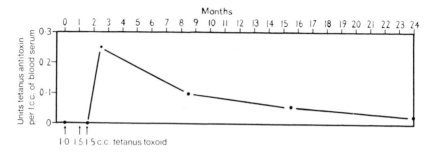

Fig. 2.5 Production of antibody as a result of three injections of tetanus toxoid (toxin rendered non-poisonous by incubation with formalin).

that we may never have suffered from clinical attacks of these diseases.

Injections of dead organisms or their toxins. The bodies of micro-organisms that have been killed contain the same chemical substances that are present in living organisms. Toxins made by growing the organisms in broth are also identical with those produced during infection. In consequence, several subcutaneous injections of suspensions of dead organisms or minute doses of toxin will stimulate the cells to produce antibodies. Because of this, the individual who has received these injections becomes immune to the organisms concerned. He may therefore escape infection if on some subsequent occasion they reach him. Employing procedures of this description we can now protect ourselves against such diseases as diphtheria, tetanus, typhoid fever and poliomyelitis.

Injection of compounds not derived from micro-organisms. In view of the fact that, fundamentally, it is a chemical compound produced by the micro-organism that stimulates the cells to produce antibodies, it is not very surprising that a series of injections of compounds having a similar type of composition, but which have not been derived from micro-organisms, may also lead to the formation of antibodies. Proteins can act in this way, so that following injections of egg white for example, antibodies are formed that react with solutions of egg white in such a way that a white insoluble precipitate is formed. But although the antibodies produced in this way are similar in every respect to those formed as a result of infection, they play no part in combating bacterial infection.

Disadvantages attending antibody production

Useful as antibodies may be in combating some infections, they may be responsible for two, fortunately rare, forms of illness.

Auto-immunization. As a general rule, the plasma cells of human beings will only produce antibodies if the substance stimulating them has come from a non-human source. But under certain conditions compounds formed in the individual's own tissues may act as antigens and stimulate the formation of antibodies and it is the combination between the antibody and the antigen that is responsible for the symptoms. Some involve only one organ such as the thyroid in Hashimoto's disease and part of the stomach in pernicious anaemia. But the process may become more widespread as in lupus erythematosus which may affect almost any part of the body.

Anaphylaxis. Human beings may from time to time receive injections of foreign substances. As a general rule, no symptoms are produced. Unfortunately, however, antibodies may be produced. If, therefore, on some subsequent occasion, a second injection of the same substance must be given, combination between this substance and antibody will occur in the tissues. This produces a very severe reaction known as *anaphylaxis*, which is probably due to the liberation of histamine into the tissues. In the more severe forms, the patient shows symptoms of shock almost before the injection is over, but in most cases there is a delay of a minute or so. The patient becomes pale and loses consciousness. There may be severe dyspnoea due to asthma and an erythematous rash accompanied by severe itching. Oedema of the face and limbs soon becomes apparent and may spread to the glottis to cause suffocation. Unless energetic treatment involving the injection of anti-histaminic drugs and adrenalin is instituted, the patient may die.

Unfortunately, sensitivity to a foreign substance can also be acquired without a previous injection and it is for this reason that some persons are sensitive to penicillin or the horse globulin that constitutes tetanus antitoxin. But such individuals can be detected because much smaller doses injected into the skin produce what is known as the *immediate-type hypersensitivity reaction* to distinguish it from another skin reaction referred to later.

Immediate-type hypersensitivity reaction. When for example a minute dose of tetanus antitoxin is injected into the skin of someone who is hypersensitive to it, the site begins to itch almost at once and within five minutes, an area of oedema surrounded by a much wider area of erythema appears. The reaction generally reaches its maximum intensity in about ten minutes. It then begins to fade and has usually disappeared within an hour. A test of this type is obviously of considerable value in clinical medicine because persons who react in this way may suffer from the potentially much more dangerous symptoms of acute anaphylaxis if larger doses are given.

Serum sickness is another manifestation of anaphylaxis. It usually occurs if a large dose of antitoxic serum has been given. No symptoms are produced at the time of injection but after an interval of 6–10 days there occurs fever, an erythematous rash with urticaria causing extreme itching, oedema of the subcutaneous tissues, pains in the joints and enlargement of lymphatic glands. The symptoms persist for a day or two and then subside. These symptoms are due to the fact that an antibody capable of reacting with the antitoxic serum is formed by the antibody-forming cells. This process takes about 6–10 days. When formed the antibody is released into the circulating blood. In this way it reaches traces of the antitoxic serum still persisting in the tissues. Combination between the two occurs and the symptoms of the disease are the result.

Cell mediated immunity

Despite a great deal of research it has never been possible to show that antibodies play any part in combating infection by certain organisms. But it is now known that another form of immunity may be responsible in which cells rather than antibodies play the predominant role. It is best exemplified by the series of events that follow inhalation of tubercle bacilli into the lungs. Here they encounter macrophages which phagocyte them as they would do with any other particulate material that reaches the lungs. But the subsequent fate of the tubercle bacilli depends on the previous history of the person who has inhaled them. If he has no immunity to tubercle bacilli, those taken up by the macrophages will survive and may even multiply. There is accordingly danger that an active infection may result. But if, on the other hand, he has acquired immunity as a result of a previous infection from which he has recovered or if he has been immunized, the tubercle bacilli do not multiply and may even die, thus averting an active infection. Once acquired, this alteration in the behaviour of the macrophages may persist as long as the individual lives.

The difference in the behaviour of the tubercle bacilli in the macrophages of immune and non-immune persons would appear to depend on the T lymphocytes. When the individual is immune, those in the vicinity of the tubercle bacilli react by producing substances that modify the behaviour of the macrophages in the way already described.

As well as rendering the patient resistant to the development of certain infections, this form of immunity also produces changes in the tissues that render them abnormally sensitive to the infecting organisms and the soluble substances produced by them in the course of growth. What part such changes play in the practical business of combating infection is still controversial. But since the skin becomes sensitive as well as other organs of the body, it is possible to detect this sensitivity by means of a very simple test. This has considerable value in medicine because it enables us to detect those who are susceptible to infection. Alternatively, it can be used diagnostically to ascertain whether or not patients are infected by certain organisms. Given the somewhat clumsy name of *delayed-type hypersensitivity reaction*, to distinguish it from another skin test referred to earlier in this chapter, it requires discussion in a little more detail.

Delayed-type hypersensitivity reaction. Many years ago, the German bacteriological pioneer, Robert Koch, found that injection of tuberculin, a substance produced by tubercle bacilli when grown in broth, into skin of a patient suffering from clinically active tuberculosis or an apparently normal person who had recovered from an attack, caused certain well marked and distinctive changes in the appearance of the skin. Nothing can be seen for 24–48 hours but an area of oedema surrounded by erythema then appears. It reaches its maximum size in three to four days and then begins to fade so that the skin becomes normal again by the end of the week. A similar dose of tuberculin injected into the skin of a normal person who has never had tuberculosis, produces no changes of any kind.

Such a test can obviously be used to detect those members of the community who have never had tuberculosis in any form and for this reason possess no immunity to the tubercle bacillus. For this purpose it is extensively employed in the form of the Mantoux and Heaf tests as a preliminary to immunization with B.C.G. vaccine. This is referred to in more detail in Chapter 7. But it can also be employed for the diagnosis of tuberculosis when the signs are equivocal. Although it is seldom used for this purpose at the present time similar reactions follow the injection of substances produced by the organisms causing brucellosis and lymphogranuloma when they are injected into the skin of patients suffering from these diseases. Skin tests of this description are therefore sometimes used for the diagnosis of such diseases.

Suppression of immunity

Up to this point, discussion has concerned the behaviour of normal persons when confronted with the organisms they encounter from time to time. These generally leave them with an increase in immunity to the organism concerned. But in view of the complicated nature of the processes that bring this about it is, perhaps, not surprising that they may sometimes fail to respond in the usual fashion. This may take several forms. The B lymphocytes, for example, may not develop into plasma cells so that antibody formation is inadequate or fails completely. In consequence, the individual is not only abnormally susceptible to the usual pathogens but to opportunistic infection by such organisms as coliform bacilli, *Proteus Pseudomonas*, and *Klebsiella* which seldom infect normal persons. Similarly, failure of the T lymphocytes to develop may lead to failure of cell mediated immunity and unusual susceptibility to tubercle bacilli and viral infection may result. If both types of lymphocyte fail to develop, susceptibility to infection becomes even greater.

Failures of this nature can be a congenital anomaly and are particularly liable to become manifest in children. But they may be brought about as a result of medication with corticosteroids in which case adults are usually involved. Cytotoxic therapy purposely applied to overcome graft rejection when organs are being transplanted may similarly depress immunity to such an extent that unusually stringent precautions must be taken to prevent infection.

3

The sources and modes of infection

In the great majority of infections, the micro-organisms only reach the patient at the start of the incubation period of the disease in question. The *source* from which they have come must, therefore, be outside the body of the patient. There must also be a *method of transmission* by which they can travel from their source to the patient. Finally, they must get into the patient by a *portal of entry*.

Much is now known of the sources, portals of entry and methods of transmission of most of the pathogenic organisms and because of this it is frequently possible to prevent infection by dealing with their sources or erecting barriers which prevent their transmission from the source to the portals of entry of human beings. Obviously, knowledge of these matters is of considerable practical importance in medicine.

THE PORTALS OF ENTRY

Organisms can enter human beings by six different routes, across the placenta, by inhalation, ingestion, implanatation, inunction and injection. Each of these must be discussed a little further.

Congenital infection across the placenta. When most

species of organisms cause infection in a pregnant women they evidently do not reach the foetus because it shows no sign that it has been infected. But some organisms may do so, particularly the spirochaete of syphilis, cytomegalovirus and the virus of german measles. In consequence, the foetus becomes infected and may die or, if born alive, may have certain specific lesions.

Inhalation. On inspiration, the air meets a series of moist surfaces in the nose, pharynx, larynx, trachea, bronchioles and lungs which abstract most of the organisms suspended in it. This is undoubtedly the mechanism by which the diphtheria bacillus, the streptococcus of scarlet fever, the meningococcus, the whooping cough bacillus, the pneumococcus, the tubercle bacillus and the viruses of measles, influenza and the common cold generally reach the respiratory tract.

Ingestion. Food or drink reaching the mouth may contain pathogenic organisms that have no action on the mucous membranes of the mouth itself or the oesophagus and stomach but which produce infection when they reach the small or large intestines.

Implantation. Under normal circumstance, the skin acts as a barrier which is impervious to most bacteria. But when the barrier is broken by accidental trauma or incision in the operating theatre, the tissues beneath become exposed. In consequence they may acquire organisms from the air, or anything that gets into the wound.

Inunction. If pathogenic organisms are present on the surface of the skin or mucous membranes, rubbing may suffice to drive them into the deeper layers and so precipitate infection. It is probably as a result of this process that boils on the neck may develop. Venereal diseases are probably transmitted by a very similar mechanism, the organisms being transferred as a result of mere contact between an area of infection and the mucous membrane that eventually becomes infected.

Injection. Biting insects such as mosquitoes and fleas may inject organisms into the deeper layers of the skin. This is the method by which yellow fever, relapsing fever and dengue are transmitted, the insect having acquired the organism from the blood of a patient it has previously bitten.

Syringes and needles used for injections may similarly convey infection. This is particularly apt to occur if they have previously been employed for abstracting blood from another person. Such blood may contain the virus of serum hepatitis and if traces still remain in the syringe or needle, this will suffice to convey infection.

THE SOURCES OF PATHOGENIC ORGANISMS

The *source* of a pathogenic organism may be defined as the situation in Nature where, under normal circumstances, it is able to survive and multiply. From such sources, the organisms may reach many other places such as the skin, clothing and bedding of human beings in the vicinity as well as dust, dirt and the surfaces of inanimate objects of all kinds. Here, they are generally unable to multiply because there is insufficient moisture and none of the foodstuffs they require. But they do not die immediately, they remain alive in a state of suspended animation. Such organisms are said to *contaminate* the surfaces they have reached while the articles on which they alighted are referred to as *vehicles*.

These terms will be used a great deal in the remainder of this chapter, for which reason it is advisable that the student has a clear idea of their meaning.

The sources of human pathogens can be divided into three categories: (1) Inanimate nature; (2) Members of the animal kingdom; and (3) Human beings themselves.

Organisms coming from inanimate nature

Many species of micro-organisms can multiply readily in substances that are not alive such as soil, dead vegetation and the bodies of animals that have died. The great majority of these organisms are quite incapable of causing human infection. The few that can do so are the bacilli responsible for tetanus, gas gangrene and botulism which may come from soil and *Proteus* which may be found in decomposing animal bodies. The same applies to *Pseudomonas*, but this organism can also survive and multiply in water. Because of this, it is common in sinks, baths and taps. It may also multiply in the water of ventilators and not only become disseminated throughout the apparatus but reach the patient to produce a particularly dangerous form of pneumonia.

Organisms coming from animals

All living things act as hosts for micro-organisms. Some may be commensals and some pathogens for the host concerned. But, on the whole, the organisms that can parasitize animals or plants are incapable of surviving, still less, causing disease in human beings. Some may be able to do so. But the type of disease caused, the animals from which the organisms come and the manner in which they reach human beings vary greatly.

Some inhabit the intestinal canal of domestic animals such as cattle, sheep, and pigs reaching the outside world in the faeces to contaminate almost everything in and around a farm. Amongst such organisms are *Pseudomonas* and *Proteus* which may reach open wounds to produce infections resembling in many respects those caused by staphylococci and streptococci. Wounds may similarly become contaminated and occasionally infected by the organisms responsible for tetanus and gas gangrene, two much more serious diseases.

Another series of organisms that may inhabit the intestinal tract of domestic animals are those responsible for food infection (*salmonellosis*). These too can reach human beings from the contaminated environment of a farm but of equal importance is the possibility that following slaughter, the intestinal contents may contaminate the meat during its preparation and if the temperature reached during cooking is not high enough human infections may result.

These micro-organisms may also inhabit the oviduct of hens and ducks and so reach the eggs before the shell has been formed. This too can be a source of human disease.

Other organisms are less widely distributed. But cows for example, may be infected by tubercle and brucellosis bacilli which are excreted in the milk and cause disease in those who drink it. Rats too may be the source of organisms pathogenic for human beings, such as those of plague and typhus which are present in the blood stream and can be conveyed to human beings by the bites of insect such as fleas or lice. Rats are also the source of the spirochaetes responsible for leptospirosis. They are excreted in the urine and so reach anyone who comes into close contact with these animals.

Parrots, pigeons and other birds may be the source of the organisms responsible for psittacosis or ornithosis, the organisms being present in the faeces. Direct contact or inhalation of the dust after it has dried can be responsible for human cases of the disease.

Other pathogenic organisms that come from animals include the viruses of yellow fever, dengue and encephalitis which are conveyed to human beings by the bites of mosquitoes and rabies derived from the saliva of a rabid animal such as a dog, cat or fox.

Organisms coming from human beings

Human beings are the only source of the great majority of the organisms that infect them. This is undoubtedly due to the fact that in the course of the centuries, such organisms have become so adapted to life as human parasites that they are unable to perpetuate their species in any other way than by growth in human beings. The human beings who act as hosts can be divided into several categories.

Patients with acute infections. In most forms of infection the organisms are present in large numbers somewhere in the patient such as the nasopharynx, lungs, intestines or wounds whence they can obtain access to the outer world in such vehicles as nasal mucus, sputum, faeces or pus and so reach other human beings. As a general rule, the organisms disappear when the patient recovers so that he can only act as a source for a comparatively short time.

Patients with chronic infections. In some diseases the infective process may last for a very long time, with the organisms continually present in the sputum, pus, etc. Tuberculosis of the lungs is perhaps the best example of this but some forms of skin infection may be equally chronic. Patients with long continued infections of this nature are obviously much more dangerous than those who have acute infections.

Convalescent carriers. In many infections of the mucous membranes, such as scarlet fever, diphtheria, typhoid fever and dysentery, the organisms may persist in the throat or intestinal canal of a small proportion of the patients for weeks or even months after the acute stage of the disease is over, and the patient appears to have made a complete recovery. The organisms usually disappear in time, but following typhoid and paratyphoid fever this may not occur and the individual becomes a permanent carrier excreting the organisms for the rest of his life.

Contact carriers. Nurses, doctors and members of the family who are in close contact with patients suffering from many forms of infection such as scarlet fever, diphtheria and dysentery, can acquire the organisms which may survive and multiply in their throats or intestinal canals for some time but without producing even mild symptoms indicative of infection. The secretions of the nasopharynx or the stools may, therefore, serve as a source of organisms for the infection of others with whom such persons come into contact. In the same way, nurses treating patients with staphylococcal infection of wounds may become nasal carriers of this organism.

Non-contact carriers. These resemble contact carriers in every respect, except that they have had no known connection with anyone who is clinically infected. In many instances, the organisms probably came from a contact carrier; but this is not invariably the case, for it is now known that some organisms may pass from non-contact carriers to normal persons to convert them into non-contact carriers in their turn. It is probably as a result of this process that many nurses in hospitals soon become carriers of penicillin-resistant strains of staphylococci.

Apparently normal persons may also carry the virus of serum hepatitis in their circulating blood. How they acquired it is unknown, but the blood of such carriers can certainly cause the disease in those who come into contact with it.

Self-contamination by cases and carriers

It has already been mentioned that organisms from an infected focus can cause infection in other persons. In this way, pus from an infected wound, a discharging sinus, or the ear in otitis media, the tears or pus coming from an infected eye, the sputum of cases of pneumonia and other infections of the lungs, or the faeces of patients with intestinal infections, may all serve as sources of pathogenic organisms.

Depending on the species of organism involved, the secretions of the nose and throat or the faeces of carriers can similarly act as sources of organisms for the infection of other persons.

It might therefore, be thought that provided the pus, sputum, tears or the faeces of infected patients and the secretions of the nose, throat or faeces of carriers, are not touched by the nurses or others in attendance, pathogenic organisms are not likely to be picked up and transferred to others. This, however, is not so, for it is now known that in addition to the infected areas of patients and the sites of multiplication on carriers, their organisms can reach other areas of their person, their clothing and their bedding. Here, they remain, sometimes for days or even weeks, in a state of suspended animation, ready as occasion offers, to pass to other persons to cause infection or convert them into carriers.

When, for example, an infected wound or discharging sinus is covered by an ordinary dressing, the organisms from the pus can apparently reach the outside of the dressings and be carried to the skin, clothing and bedding. This is well illustrated in Figure 3.1 which shows the situations to which staphylococci from purulent infections may, apparently, travel. There are, it

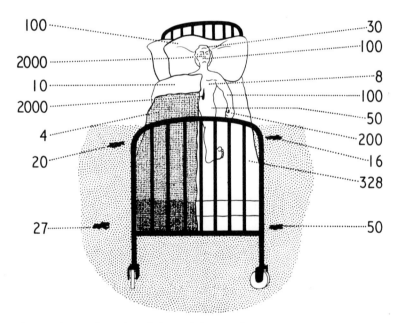

Fig. 3.1 The number of staphylococci that may be present on different areas of the skin, bedding and floor when a patient has a staphylococcal infection of a wound.

is true, considerable variations in the extent to which this occurs, but it is obvious that it can be very widespread indeed. It will also be observed that the lower sheet of the bed is frequently contaminated. This means that it would be impossible to make the bed of such a patient without the hands of the nurse becoming contaminated.

If the patient has an intestinal infection, there is similar danger that his organisms may reach his skin or his bedding. This is particularly liable to occur with children who defaecate into napkins.

Carriers too, may have their own organisms on many parts of their skin and clothing, some of which may be a considerable distance from the area of the body in which they are multiplying. Staphylococci, for example, come from the nose. This, with most persons, is the only part of the body where they actually multiply. But they may be carried, probably by the fingers, to many other parts of the body. Figure 3.2 illus-

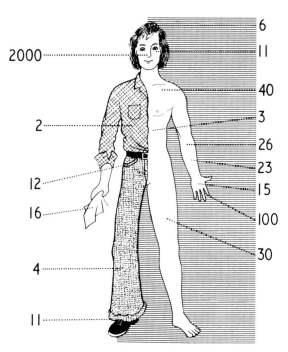

Fig. 3.2 The number of staphylococci that may be present on different areas of the skin and clothing of a nasal carrier.

trates the areas most likely to be contaminated in this way. Such organisms are only seldom found on these areas if the individual is not a carrier.

Estimates of the actual number of organisms on the skin and clothing of carriers show that some carriers may have a great many. But there is no doubt that the largest number likely to be encountered is on the fingers. The palms, wrists and forearms are much less heavily contaminated. This is probably because they do not come directly into contact with the nose.

When the carrier has pathogenic organisms in his faeces, they may reach his own fingers every time he defaecates. For ordinary lavatory paper is sufficiently porous to allow some of them to pass through.

Thus, although the organisms from a carrier may come from his nose, throat or faeces, there is no doubt whatever that they may also be present on many other parts of his body as well.

Self-contamination in this way is obviously of very great importance because it means that whether the patient is suffering from some form of infection or is a symptomless carrier, he is a much more dangerous individual than might be thought. For his organisms are by no means confined to the infected area or the carrier site.

METHODS BY WHICH MICRO-ORGANISMS ARE TRANSMITTED FROM THEIR SOURCES TO THEIR PORTALS OF ENTRY

From what has already been said, it should be obvious that whatever their real source may be, most pathogenic organisms must travel some distance in the outer world in a state of suspended animation, from their source to the portal of entry of their next victim. To a large extent, the distance travelled, the route followed, and the time taken to do so, depend on the organism involved.

Perhaps the most extreme example of this is the bacillus that causes anthrax. Wool coming to this country from another as far distant as Indonesia, may have been derived from an animal with the disease and be heavily contaminated by the spores of this organism. When therefore, the bales of wool reach this country, these spores may reach the men unpacking them and produce the typical malignant pustule on the skin or wool sorters' pneumonia if they are inhaled. In this instance, the distance between the real source of the organisms and the patient who becomes infected is many thousands of miles, and the occurence of infection is, to large extent, due to the fact that the spores that convey the disease are so highly resistant that they can survive long sea voyages. The gonococcus on the other hand, is a very different organism. It produces gonorrhoea and is so easily killed by drying and exposure to oxygen that it cannot survive for more than an hour or so, once it has left the genital tract. In consequence, it cannot travel any distance and it is probably for this reason that gonorrhoea can, as a general rule, be only acquired as a result of direct contact with an infected area.

Other organisms lie between these two extremes, most of them being able to remain alive in a state of suspended animation for some time after leaving the tissues of the case or carrier from whom they have been derived.

Thus the particular pathway along which an organism travels from its source to its victims may be very long or very short. It may, it should be added, be as tortuous as a Devonshire lane or as direct as a motorway. But whatever its length and however devious it may be, it is a matter of very considerable importance that we have some idea of the sources of pathogenic organisms and the routes by which they travel, because, as is shown in Chapters 4 and 5, it is frequently possible to prevent the spread of infection by a particular micro-organism if we can introduce measures that eliminate its sources or cut its lines of communication. The remainder of this chapter is, accordingly, devoted to a discussion of the usual sources of micro-organisms and the lines of communication by which they travel.

Infections of the respiratory tract

Many different organisms infect the respiratory tract. Some, such as the viruses of measles and smallpox, produce widespread catarrhal infection in the mouth, nose and pharynx which may even extend into the bronchi and lungs. But most organisms tend to infect more circumscribed areas so that the viruses of the common cold generally attack the nose and pharynx; the diphtheria bacillus and haemolytic streptococcus are more likely to grow on the tonsils and fauces; while the whooping cough bacillus infects the bronchi and the pneumococcus, one or more lobes of the lung.

There seems to be little doubt that in all these diseases the organisms generally enter the patient in the air he breathes and are deposited on the mucous membrane of the area which eventually becomes infected.

Sources

The organisms responsible for infections in these areas are almost invariably derived from human beings. The two exceptions, are psittacosis, a form of pneumonia whose virus comes from parrots, and wool sorters' disease, another variety of pneumonia which may follow the inhalation of the spores of the anthrax bacillus liberated into the atmosphere from the wool of infected sheep.

Human beings who act as the sources of the organisms may themselves be in the acute stage of the disease with the organisms present in large numbers in the nasal secretions, saliva

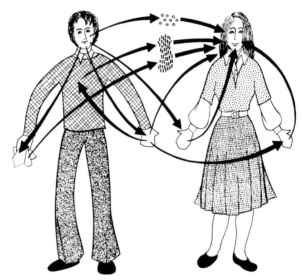

Fig. 3.3 Routes by which organisms infecting the nose or throat may be transmitted from person to person.

or sputum. But they may also be present in the noses or throats of convalescent, contact or non-contact carriers and there is no doubt that such individuals are responsible for many cases of diphtheria, scarlet fever and whooping cough and, in all probability, influenza and common colds. But symptomless carriers of the viruses of measles and smallpox are unknown.

Method of transmission

To a very large extent the transmission of respiratory organisms depends on the type of individual who acts as their source. When he is producing large quantities of sputum brought up in paroxysms of coughing, there can be little doubt that the organisms that are known to be present in the larger particles are able to travel quite long distances through the atmosphere. In this way, they may be conveyed directly to the mouth or nose of someone in the vicinity.

But in many infections, little, if any, sputum is produced, while carriers generally produce none, neither do they cough. In spite of this, however, their organisms may still reach other persons. The mechanism by which this takes place is still controversial. There are two theories.

One, the oldest, postulates that person to person transmission occurs by organisms present in droplets that issue from the mouth or nose when speaking, coughing or sneezing. There are, however, serious objections to this theory. In the first place, very few of the droplets come from the nose even when sneezing, the great majority consisting of particles of saliva from the front of the mouth. Secondly, with the possible exception of measles and smallpox, this saliva contains very few pathogens even when there is an acute infection of the nose or throat, for which reason, very few of the droplets will contain them. Thirdly, the behaviour of the droplets themselves does not facilitate their reaching another person easily. For the larger droplets that contain whatever pathogens are likely to be expelled, fall so rapidly to the ground out of harm's way as soon as they leave the mouth that only under very exceptional circumstances will they reach another person. The smaller droplets may however, remain suspended as 'droplet nuclei' and can be carried long distances by air currents. They may, accordingly reach another person. But very few, if any, contain pathogenic organisms.

Thus despite the widespread belief that talking, coughing and above all, sneezing convey respiratory infection, it is most improbable that they play any but a minor role.

It is much more probable that organisms are conveyed by another mechanism altogether. Whether the donor is actively infected or is only a carrier, he will touch his nose or lips a great many times in the course of a day. As a result, both his fingers and handkerchief will become contaminated by organisms in the nose or mouth. The pillow and bedclothes will similarly become contaminated during the night and his face cloth and towel every time he washes. Because of this, nasal mucus and saliva, together with any organisms in them will quickly become dispersed over his skin, clothing, bedding and other objects in his vicinity.

The secretions will quickly dry leaving some at least of the organisms alive on these surfaces. They can then get to another person in three different ways. The nose or mouth of the latter may touch them when kissing for example. Secondly, the fingers of the recipient may touch the contaminated surfaces and convey the organisms to his own nose or mouth. But the third method is probably the most important. This depends on the fact that whenever the skin, clothing, bedding, etc., are rubbed, shaken or disturbed in any way, minute particles consisting of scales from the skin, or fluff and dust from the clothing and bedding are released into the atmosphere in the neighbourhood. They may then be conveyed long distances by air currents. Any organisms that have contaminated the surfaces from which they have come will accompany them. As a result, they may be inhaled by anyone nearby and so reach his respiratory tract.

Intestinal infections

The commonest form of intestinal infection is the acute diarrhoea and vomiting that may follow the consumption of food containing one or other of the bacilli of food infection. This is usually referred to as food poisoning. Acutally this is usually due to growth of organisms in the intestines and not to poisons present in the food. For this reason infections of this nature will be referred to in this book as food infection.

Dysentery is another form of intestinal infection in which severe diarrhoea is the most prominent symptom. A third disease is cholera in which there may be severe purgation and vomiting.

Typhoid and paratyphoid fevers are also intestinal infections but there is much less tendency to diarrhoea. Indeed the principal symptoms are due to invaion of the blood stream by the organisms. Poliomyelitis is another intestinal infection and this is the only manifestation in many cases, but the virus may travel to the spinal cord to produce the paralyses which are characteristic of the disease.

Sources

In general, human beings are the sources from which these organisms are derived. They may be patients who are already infected or they may be carriers.

The organisms are certainly present in large numbers in the faeces during the acute stage of all these diseases and except following cholera, they frequently continue to be excreted for some considerable time during convalescence. Convalescent carriers may therefore be the source of the organisms. In time, the organisms cease to be excreted, but following typhoid or paratyphoid fever, some patients may become permanent carriers who excrete these organisms for the rest of their lives. Some of them may also excrete them in the urine.

Individuals with atypical infections can be equally dangerous. They may have such mild and transient symptoms that the real nature of their illness may not be suspected. But they may not only excrete the organisms in their faeces during this phase of their illness, but continue to do so for weeks or even months after all symptoms have disappeared.

Normal persons living in close proximity to patients with both fully developed and atypical infections, may also acquire the organims and become contact carriers. They too excrete the organisms in the faeces and may continue to do so for some time.

However, some intestinal infections are derived not from other human beings but from animals. Salmonella infection, a common cause of disease in man, is spread in this way.

Organisms present in the bowel of the animal contaminate the flesh and are present on raw meat brought into the kitchen. If the food is inadequately cooked or if the organisms are allowed to get into contact with cooked food, the possibility of infection of people eating the food exists, particularly if the food is kept at a temperature at which the organisms can multiply. Outbreaks of food infection due to salmonellas have often been traced to foods such as chickens and pies.

Intestinal pathogens may also be present in shellfish, particularly those taken from the water of estuaries into which the drainage of large cities can find access.

Method of transmission

Except when they have come from shellfish, animals or birds, the organisms undoubtedly reach human beings in such vehicles as food or drink that have become contaminated as a result of transfer of the organisms from the faeces of cases or carriers. Usually, the organisms do not multiply in the vehicles by which they are conveyed, but when they reach milk, this does occur. Contaminated milk can, therefore, be very dangerous.

Whether or not the vehicles will become contaminated by organisms from the faeces of patients or carriers, depends to a very large extent on the methods employed for the disposal of faeces and urine.

In extremely primitive communities, where there is virtually no knowledge of hygiene, organisms in the faeces of a patient with a disease such as cholera, typhoid or dysentery may reach the hands of the attendants and be carried directly to food or water and the vessels containing them. In this way, they can easily reach other members of the household. Even when this does not occur, the organisms can still reach others if the faeces are deposited on the ground outside or into a shallow latrine. Thence, they may be washed by rain into the pond, stream or well from which the inhabitants obtain their water for drinking or the preparation of vegetables or fruit that are consumed without cooking. Alternatively, faecal organisms may be carried on the feet of flies which are invariably attracted to faeces, and so reach food or the vessels in which it is served in neighbouring houses. In hot, dry climates, dust from dried

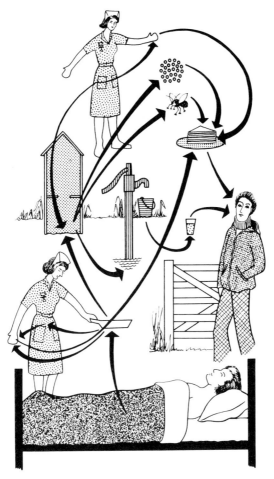

Fig. 3.4 Routes by which organisms present in the faeces of a carrier (upper left) or a patient (lower right) may reach another individual.

faeces may likewise carry faecal organisms into houses and on to unprotected food or water.

When the organisms come from carriers, they follow the same routes. But carriers are less dangerous than patients, partly because they do not suffer from the diarrhoea with numerous liquid stools which is a common event in most intestinal infections, and partly because fewer pathogens are present in their faeces than in those of patients in the acute stage of infection.

In more advanced communities which employ buckets, privies or cesspools for the disposal of excreta, there is the same danger of transfer of the organisms to food or crockery in the household, and that flies or dust may carry the organisms into it from the places where the faeces have been deposited. There is also danger that the organisms from privies or cesspools may be able to reach the water supply. This is particularly liable to occur if the water comes from a shallow well because it can be contaminated by pathogenic organisms that have been carried through the soil from a nearby privy or cesspool. Water taken from a stream or pond may also be contaminated if a cesspool in the neighbourhood has been allowed to overflow so that its contents are able to reach the water.

In the most civilized communities, extremely efficient methods for the disposal of faeces and urine are employed. They are deposited directly into a water closet and carried by a stream of water in underground drains to sewage disposal plants where all the pathogenic organisms are removed from the sewage by the activities of other species of micro-organisms. Nevertheless, even when the most up to date apparatus is employed, there is still some danger that pathogenic organisms may reach others.

Carriers can, for example, contaminate their own fingers every time they defaecate. For it is known that the pathogenic organisms in their faeces can pass through the ordinary lavatory paper and get on to their fingers. This is particularly apt to occur if the stools are liquid. Once the fingers are contaminated, the organisms can only too easily reach foodstuffs, fruit and vegetables the carrier may subsequently prepare for consumption by others. This is a method by which typhoid and paratyphoid fever may be acquired.

The bedpan that must be employed by hospital patients may also prove to be a source of infection for while it is being emptied in the sluice room, it is virtually impossible to avoid splashing. If, therefore, the patient is a carrier, and still more so if he is actually infected, pathogenic organisms may reach both the hands and the uniform of the nurse. Transfer of the organisms to food may then occur unless the hands are carefully washed.

Babies' napkins can be equally dangerous, for it is impossible to remove one that is soiled without faeces reaching the hands and sometimes, the uniform.

Gastro-enteritis in infancy

Children in the first year of life are liable to an acute intestinal disease characterized by diarrhoea and vomiting with, in the more severe cases, extreme dehydration. There seems to be little doubt that these symptoms are due to infection but what variety of organism is responsible is still a controversial matter. There is evidence that many of these infections are due to certain strains of coliform bacilli that are more pathogenic than others. But there is also an increasing body of evidence that viruses may cause similar symptoms. Breast-fed infants are much less likely to suffer from gastro-enteritis than are those that are bottle-fed.

Children living at home may become infected but at least in developed countries, it is more usual for the disease to occur in hospitals, usually in the form of epidemics amongst new-born babies or somewhat older children in paediatric wards.

Sources

Although an adult carrier may be responsible for introducing the disease into a nursery it is more probable that the source is another child coming to the nursery with little or no sign of clinical infection.

Method of transmission

It is extrmely probable that the hands of the nurse are the principal factors in the transmission of these organisms because they can be contaminated by her own faecal organisms if she herself is a carrier or those in the napkins of infected children she has handled. The organisms may then reach the teats, the food itself or the bottles into which it is put. In support of this there is evidence that under poor hygienic conditions, these infections are commoner amongst children receiving artificial food than those who are breast fed.

Infection of wounds

Whenever the continuity of the skin is broken by some form of injury, the tissues beneath are exposed to micro-organisms on the object that caused the wound or that may be present in its immediate environment. The great majority of these organisms are not pathogenic and are quickly dealt with by the defence mechanisms in the wounded area, but several different varieties of organisms may be able to resist them and so survive to cause infection.

The most usual form of infection involves the formation of pus and such infections are usually referred to as pyogenic. But another series of organisms, known as the spore-bearing anaerobes, can also enter wounds to produce the very different signs and symptoms of gas gangrene or tetanus. These are discussed in a separate section (see p. 68).

Organisms responsible.

The most dangerous are haemolytic streptococci. Not only do they produce severe inflammatory changes in the tissues of the wound itself but the organisms tend to spread to the deeper tissues and by way of the lymphatics to the regional lymph nodes. They may also invade the blood stream to be carried to vital organs such as the lungs or brain where metastatic infections that may kill the patient may be the result.

Staphylococci are much more likely to produce infection of wounds but the infection itself is generally less severe for they seldom invade the deeper tissues or reach the lymph glands or blood stream. Recovery usually occurs but healing of the wound is delayed.

Pseudomonas, Proteus and coliform bacilli may also cause wound infections which are seldom severe and recovery is the rule.

Sources

Most of the organisms that cause wound infections come from human beings who are either suffering from some form of infection or are symptomless carriers.

Infected individuals. Open wounds that have already become infected are important sources of the organisms for they are not only present in the wound itself but also in the dressings and on the skin in the vicinity. But wounds vary greatly in this respect; an extensive burn or scald being obviously much more dangerous than a cut or abrasion.

Naturally occurring infections that have nothing to do with injury constitute a second possible source. Pus from pimples, boils, styes, paronychiae and impetigo or from deeper infections that have been incised such as abscesses, carbuncles and cellulitis are examples.

Carriers. All the organisms responsible for wound infections can persist, sometimes for long periods, in the bodies of symptomless carriers. Staphylococci for example, are normal inhabitants of the anterior part of the nose or the skin of the perineum of a high proportion of the human population. Carriers of haemolytic streptococci are not so common but about 7 per cent have them in the throat and 1 per cent in the nose. *Pseudomonas, Proteus* and coliform bacilli are frequently present in the faeces of normal persons and these too constitute another source of organisms.

It is thus obvious that the organisms capable of causing infection of wounds can not only come from a whole series of different forms of infectinfection, but are common inhabitants of the tissues of normal persons as well. With such an abundance of sources, it is perhaps surprising that any wound succeeds in escaping infection.

Method of transmission

There being no reason to suppose that the organisms responsible for infection of wounds are already present in the tissues before the wound is inflicted, it follows that the organisms must get into it either at the moment of infliction or during the subsequent period before it is finally healed.

Organisms introduced at the time of infliction. It is most improbable that the organisms that cause wound infections are at all common on the objects that usually cause traumatic wounds. Few will survive for very long on wood, metal or glass and even fewer on the heated objects and boiling water that cause burns and scalds. Foreign bodies that may be forced into the wounds at the time of infliction such as stones, dirt and dust are unlikely to be contaminated by the more dangerous organisms such as streptococci and staphylococci but *Pseudomonas, Proteus* and coliform bacilli may be present because they are common in faeces. On the other hand, particles of

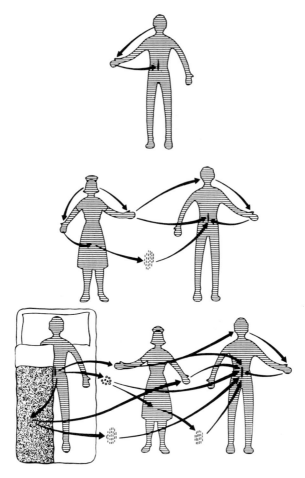

Fig. 3.5 Some of the routes by which staphylococci and streptococci may reach open wounds. Top figure, organisms coming from the patient's own nose or throat. Centre figure, organisms coming from a carrier. Lower figure, organisms coming from another patient with an already infected wound.

skin or clothing are potentially at least, more dangerous because they may be contaminated by any of the organisms that cause infection of wounds if the victim is a carrier.

Wounds produced by incision in the operating theatre or outpatient's department are in a very different category. They are invariably produced by carefully sterilized instruments and the skin through which the incision is made has been washed and treated with antiseptics. Even if the individual is a carrier, any organisms present on his skin have probably been killed or removed by these procedures. However, organisms present in the patient's bowel may contaminate the wound if the bowel is opened during the course of surgery. This is difficult to prevent and it is for this reason that short courses of antibiotics are now often given to prevent wound infection.

Organisms introduced after infliction. There is a great deal of evidence that the organisms may reach both traumatic and operation wounds at almost any time between their infliction and healing. They can do this in at least four different ways.

1. They may come from the nose, throat or faeces of the patient himself. Although there seems to be no doubt that infection of wounds can occur as a result of this process, it must be confessed that very little is known of the route followed by the organisms.
2. They may come from a carrier attending the wound who has the organisms in his nose or throat. It is however extremely improbable that, except in quite unusual circumstance, they are ever propelled directly into the wound. Their transfer is more likely to occur by indirect methods which are detailed below.
   (a) Since the organisms may be on the fingers of the carrier, they can reach the wound during its treatment if the bare hands are used to explore it, clean it, insert stitches, palpate the skin in the vicinity or remove the dressing. Even when gloves are worn, there is still danger that the organisms may reach the wound through minute holes that have not been detected.
   (b) The organisms are also present on the skin or clothing of the carrier. They will remain there so long as he remains still. But movement of any kind will dislodge them into the atmosphere roundabout. Walking, movement of the arms or agitation of the clothing will serve. Dissemination of organisms in this way can still occur in operating theatres despite the wearing of a sterile gown and gloves. As a result of these forms of activity, the organisms may be carried in air currents into the wound while it is exposed. But it is of considerable interest that women are much less likely to disperse organisms from the skin than men.

3. They may come from a surgeon or nurse who is suffering from an apparently trivial infection such as stye, or a boil. Very little is known of the route followed by the organisms but there seems to be no doubt that infections on the arm are the most dangerous.
4. They may come from a patient in a neighbouring bed who has an infected wound, skin infection, discharging abscess or sinus or an infection of the respiratory tract, to reach a hitherto uninfected wound in a variety of ways.
   (a) They may contaminate the hands of an attendant who touches the infected area and then without washing or other treatment, dresses another wound.
   (b) They may contaminate a bath, basin or toilet article which is subsequently used by another patient with an open wound.
   (c) They may be released on minute particles into the atmosphere whenever the dressings covering an infected area are disturbed in any way. Such particles may reach an open wound in a nearby bed directly by air currents or by carriage on the nurse's hands. But they may also do so by an indirect route whose first step is contamination of the skin on the rest of the patient's body, his bedding and the floor in the vicinity. The second step is any form of disturbance such as making the bed or sweeping the floor which liberates some of the infected particles into the atmosphere where they may be carried by air currents to a neighbouring bed.

It is thus obvious that the organisms that cause infection of wounds may come from many different sources and be carried to the wounds in a variety of ways.

Tetanus

This is a severe infection and may cause the death of the patinet. The disease is due to the growth of the tetanus bacilli in the wound but the severe symptoms—spasms or convulsions which may involve the whole body—are due to the formation by the organism of an exotoxin which acts on the central nervous system. Tetanus is an anaerobic organism, that is it is unable to multiply in the presence of oxygen. For this reason although the spores of tetanus bacilli are often found in wounds they seldom germinate.

Tetanus bacilli are found in the bowel of many animals particularly cattle and horses and they reach the soil of farms and gardens in manure. The highly resistant spores may of remain alive for many years and soil is therefore an important source of the organism. If tetanus spores are introduced into a wound at the time it is infected and if the conditions in the wound allow the spores to germinate tetanus will result. It is becoming an uncommon disease in developed countries due to widespread immunisation.

Gas gangrene

This is also a serious disease and like tetanus is caused by an anaerobic spore-forming organism. However, in the case of gas gangrene the source of the organism is the patient's own bowel. Gas gangrene is most commonly seen following amputation of the leg when this is carried out because of a poor blood supply. If the remaining tissue is still poorly oxygenated gas gangrene may result. The disease gets it name because gas is formed in the tissues but there are other more serious generalised consequences of the disease which if untreated are fatal.

Infections of the bladder and urinary tract

Cystitis and pyelonephritis are usually due to coliform bacilli, *Proteus* or *Pseudononas* which are probably derived from the intestinal canal of the patient himself. Their ability to cause such infections is largely due to the fact that they can multiply in urine. It is for this reason that these organisms may also cause infection of the bladder or operation wound when it is necessary to drain the bladder following prostatectomy. For if they are able to reach the urine in the drainage bottle or plastic bag that is sometimes used, they may multiply in it, reach the tubing connecting it with the patient and grow along the urine in the tubing to reach the bladder and so set up infection.

Nor is this the only danger. Once these organisms have contaminated an ordinary urinal, drainage bottle or plastic container, they will persist in them until they are sterilized. Unless this precaution has been taken, any urine subsequently deposited in them provides an ideal culture medium for the organisms. For this reason unsterilized urine containers should not be used in genito-urinary wards.

Infections of the liver

On the whole, the liver is only seldom the site of an active infection but in tropical countries it may be seriously damaged by the virus of yellow fever which generally reaches it by way of the blood stream from the bite of a mosquito infected from another patient with the disease. The spirochaetes responsible for leptospirosis may also cause ifnection in the liver. They are present in the urine of rats and other animals and although they can enter by way of cuts and scratches infection is also possible if they are swallowed.

Of more importance in other parts of the world is hepatitis A or epidemic jaundice. The virus is present in the faeces during the acute stage of the disease and can reach others by the same routes as those followed by other intestinal organisms.

The second form of the disease is hepatitis B or serum hepatitis. It is fortunately rare, the symptoms may be more severe and death more probable. But epidemiologically it is very different. The virus is present in the circulating blood of a small proportion of the population to whom it does no harm. But the blood is the main vehicle by which it is conveyed to other persons. Traces left in needles, on instruments or in flasks and tubing may suffice. More recently, the blood left in the apparatus employed in operating theatres and dialysis units has come under suspicion but thanks to the precautions taken, few cases now occur.

Infections of the meninges

The meninges may become infected by pyogenic organisms if the skull is fractured permitting their access to the cerebrospinal fluid. A second way in which the meninges may become infected is as a result of direct spread from mastoid cells that have become infected by pneumococci from the middle ear. But the meningococcus and *Haemophilus* can cause meningitis by an entirely different process. These organisms may be present in the nose of carriers and are disseminated from person to person in much the same way as are other organisms of the respiratory tract. They may then reach the blood stream and when this occurs, they tend to settle in the meninges to cause meningitis. A similar infection can also be caused by the pneumococcus.

Infections of the skin, hair and conjuctiva

Several organisms may produce infection of the skin. Staphylococci for example, are responsible for furunculosis, styes, boils, carbuncles and one form of impetigo. There is now a great deal of evidence that the organisms responsible have generally come from the nose of the patient himself and have probably been conveyed to the site of infection by his fingers or handkerchief.

Streptococcal infections are less common. In erysipelas, the deeper layers of the skin are involved but in impetigo (which may also be caused by this organism) it is more superficial. But in both, the organisms have probably come from the nose or throat of the patient himself.

A very unusual infection of the skin is the malignant pustule of anthrax. This is generally the result of contact with an infected animal such as an ox or a sheep. The wool or hide may also be contaminated by the organism and produce infection in those who handle them.

Fungi may also cause infections of the skin. The most usual is athlete's foot or tinea pedis which is usually contracted as a result of walking barefooted in communal bathing places such as sports clubs or the showers installed for miners at pit heads.

In tropical countries that have a hot moist climate, fungal infections of the skin (but which may invade deeper tissues as well) are commoner than in temperate climates. Sporotrichosis and Madura foot are two examples and in both instances the fungi probably get into the skin from the soil where, thanks to the warmth and moisture, the organisms responsible have been able to survive and multiply.

The hair itself is not as a rule likely to be infected by the usual pathogenic organisms. But certain species of fungi can do so and cause ringworm, in which the hair becomes so brittle that it breaks, leaving bald patches. The organisms may come from other human beings and are generally transferred as a result of close contact with other cases of the disease. It is therefore common in schools. Other species may, however, come from domestic animals such as cattle, dogs and cats.

Many different species of organism can cause conjunctivitis. Epidemics of 'pink eye' that occur in schools and similar institutions are probably due to transfer of the organisms in tears or pus to others by way of towels, pillows and similar objects. Another form of conjunctivitis known as 'shipyard eye' and due to a virus, has been shown to be due to the transfer of the organisms on pipettes used for dropping solutions into eyes.

Lastly, mention must be made of trachoma an extremely important disease because of its tendency to produce blindness. It usually starts in infancy as an infection of the upper eyelid. Common in developing countries such as Egypt and China, there seems no doubt that its high prevalence is largely due to disregard of even elementary hygiene, it being spread by flies, dirty clothing and unwashed hands.

Puerperal infections

Infections of the uterus after delivery may be comparatively trivial and without any clear evidence that any particular organism is responsible. But the severe cases are nearly always due to either haemolytic streptococci or to anaerobic streptococci.

Those due to haemolytic streptococci are generally the result of transfer of the organisms from throat or nose carriers amongst the attendants at the time of delivery. They probably reach the birth canal by way of the fingers. Cross infection from other cases can occur, but is nowadays very unusual.

The causation of anaerobic streptococcal infections is entirely different. These organisms are already present in the vagina of many women before delivery and when infection occurs, it is nearly always due to transfer of these organisms to the cervix or placental site. This is particularly likely to occur if the delivery is complicated in any way.

Staphylococcal infections of new-born children

Children in hospital nurseries are particularly liable to staphylococcal infections of the conjunctiva, breast and skin. It is probable that the particular strain of staphylococcus responsible is introduced into the nursery by a nurse or midwife who is either a carrier or who has some form of superficial infection such as a boil or a stye. Her fingers will probably be contaminated so that the organism reaches one or other of the babies she attends. In this way it reaches the nose or the raw surface of the umbilical stump where it survives and multiplies without necessarily producing signs or symptoms of an active infection. In this way a number of babies may become nasal and umbilical carriers within a few hours of birth (see Fig. 3.6).

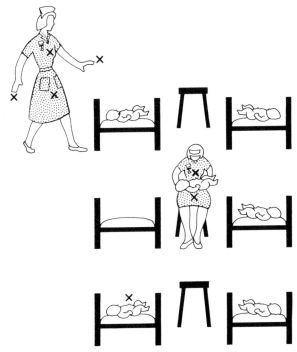

Fig. 3.6 Transmission of straphylococci from a nurse who is a nasal carrier to an newborn baby.

Once introduced into the nursery in this way, the organism reaches every new-born baby in turn. This probably occurs in a variety of ways; from baby to baby by the nurse's fingers or uniform which have been contaminated by contact with a baby who is a carrier (see Fig. 3.7) or by airborne particles contami-

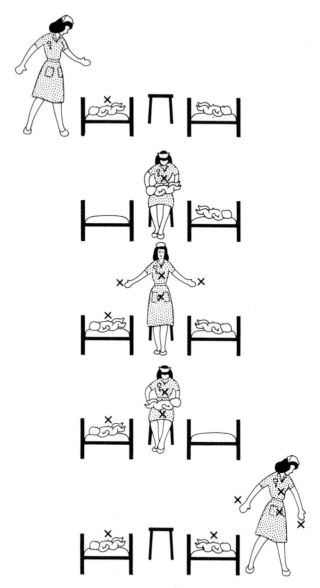

Fig. 3.7 Transmission of staphylococci from the umbilicus of a baby to another baby by a nurse who is not a nasal carrier.

nated by staphylococci released from the clothing or bedding or carrier babies.

If the strain introduced into the nursery in this way is sufficiently pathogenic, some of the babies may become infected.

Venereal infections

Syphilis and gonorrhoea are nearly always spread from person to person in course of the sexual act. But they may, rarely, be transmitted by contamination of objects such as bedding, lavatories or towels. Gonococcal vulvo-vaginitis has also occurred in the form of small epidemics in children living under very poor hygienic conditions.

Insect-borne diseases

In communities where faeces are deposited on the ground or in unprotected privies or buckets, pathogenic organisms such as those of enteric and dysentery may be coveyed to the food or drink of other individuals by house-flies. In this, insects merely act as mechanical conveyors whereas the organisms causing other forms of infection not only depend entirely on insects for transmission, but the organism must actually multiply in the body of the insect. Such insects are frequently referred to as *vectors*.

Different species of insect take part in this process and as a general rule, the organisms causing each disease can only be transmitted by the appropriate species of insect. Because of this, many of the diseases referred to below are only found in countries where the climate is suitable for the development of the insect concerned.

Mosquitoes. A species of mosquito that will only develop in hot climates, known as *Aëdes aegypti*, conveys the viruses of yellow fever and dengue from human being to human being. A number of other species transmit the viruses causing encephalitis from the animals or birds which are their true hosts to human being.

Whether the viruses come from Man or animals, they are present in their circulating blood and accordingly reach the gut of the mosquito when it abstracts blood. The viruses then develop in the body cells and ultimately reach the salivary glands. This process takes time. In the case of yellow fever and dengue, development of the viruses in *Adës aegypti* requires 11–12 days and during this period the mosquito cannot transmit them. But once this phase is over the mosquito remains capable of doing so for the remainder of its life. This is effected by injection of some of the virus present in the saliva into the wound when the insect bites a susceptible individual.

Fleas. Fleas are responsible for the transmission of some diseases, the most important of which is plague. The organism is a natural pathogen of the rat and when the latter becomes infected the bacilli are present in enormous numbers in the circulating blood. When, therefore, the fleas that usually infest rats take blood which is their only nourishment, the organisms are caught up in the clots that form when the blood coagulates in their intestinal tracts. These multiply rapidly and eventually form a solid mass of plague bacilli occupying most of the stomach and foregut.

Under normal circumstances, rat fleas do not bite human beings but if, as generally occurs, most of the rats die of their infection, the fleas become sufficiently hungry to transfer their attention to human beings who may be in the vicintiy. They accordingly attempt to abstract blood, but the plague bacilli in their foregut act rather like a ball valve and prevent entry of the blood into the stomach. In their efforts to overcome this impediment, the fleas regurgitate some of the organisms into the skin. The plague bacilli then travel along the lymphatics to the lymph glands where they are caught up and begin to multiply. The inflammatory process causes swelling of the gland. Such a gland is known as a bubo and this form of the disease is usually referred to as bubonic plague. In some cases, the organisms may reach the blood stream from their portal of entry to produce a generalized infection or septicaemic plague.

Lice. Lice are not usually found on the bodies of human beings who possess the necessary facilities for keeping themselves clean. But when it becomes impossible to obtain soap, hot water and a change of clothing, they almost always become infested by lice. These insects require human blood as food, and obtain it by puncturing the skin. This causes irritation but need not produce disease.

If however the organisms responsible for certain diseases

such as relapsing fever, and epidemic typhus, are present in the circulating blood, they reach the intestinal canal of the louse. They then enter the cells lining the intestinal canal where they start to multiply; after 7–14 days they leave the cells and are excreted by the louse in its faeces.

While this is taking place, the patient on whom the louse is parasitic may have died of the infection and when this occurs, the louse, if it is to survive, must find another human being from whom to obtain blood. If it succeeds in reaching some other person it will not only take blood but defaecate on to his skin. Because of the irritation, the individual who has acquired the louse will scratch the area and in so doing may rub some of the organisms into his skin. In this way they reach the circulating blood and in due course produce the disease.

Other insects. Little need be said about the remaining insect vectors responsible for conveying other forms of infection to human beings. Sandflies convey sandfly fever. Mites transmit the causative agent of scrub typhus and the viruses of certain forms of encephalitis from a variety of animal hosts to man. Ticks are responsible for the transmission of the viruses of other forms of encephalitis as well as the agents responsible for African relapsing fever, and Rocky Mountain spotted fever. In all these instances the organisms come from the animals which are their true hosts.

CROSS INFECTION

As described in the preceding pages, many of the organisms that cause human infections are derived from other human beings who are either already infected or are symptomless carriers. As a result, some of those acquiring these organisms may, in their turn, become clinically infected or harbour the organisms as contact carriers. Theoretically, this process can occur anywhere but since it necessitates some form of contact with other people, much depends on the type of community involved. If, for example, it is in the depths of the country with the inhabitants living in scattered farmsteads or small hamlets, they may meet each other so seldom that person to person transmission of organisms may occur only seldom. But if they live and particularly sleep in close knit communities such as a hospital, residential school or college, the barracks of an army unit or the crew quarters of a ship, there will be many apportunities for the person to person transmission of organisms and the production of disease. It is the process that is usually referred to as *cross infection.*

As a result, such viruses as those of poliomyelitis, measles and influenza and the haemolytic streptococci of tonsillitis and scarlet fever may produce quite severe outbreaks in communities of this nature. Staphylococci too, can behave in this way for they can be readily transferred from nose to nose of normal persons, thence to wounds to produce infections and then, in the reverse direction, from infected wounds to the noses of other patients or the nurses in attendance. But although the dissemination of staphylococci and particularly those that are resistant to antibiotics, is frequently stressed in hospitals so much that it would be pardonable to assume that this is all that cross infection implies, it must be emphasized that this is not the case for it is but part of a general phenomenon that can occur in communities of different kinds and caused by many different organisms.

Hospital acquired infection

Although the patients and staff in hospitals may become infected as a result of cross infection, it may also come to them from sources and by processes that have nothing to do with cross infection. For this reason, the portmanteau term *hospital acquired infection* has recently been introduced to include not only cross infection but infections acquired in other ways. Perhaps the best example is infection by *Pseudomonas.* Being able to multiply in water and unaffected by some antiseptics, it may be present in supposedly sterile water, in humidifier bottles and even in antiseptic solutions. In such situations, it may cause ifnection of wounds, the lungs or the eyes. A second example is food infection caused by organisms already present in meat or eggs at the time of their arrival in the hospital kitchen. Under certain circumstances such organisms may not be killed in the cooking process or, alternatively may reach the food after it has been cooked. In all these instances, the organisms undoubtedly reach the patient from somewhere in the hospital but not by what is usually understood as cross infection.

*Procedures at ports
and frontiers
Procedures within the
country*

4

Prevention of infection by control of the sources of micro-organisms

It is a cardinal principle in medicine that it is generally easier and much more desirable to prevent disease than allow it to develop and then cure it. Many diseases still cannot be prevented but those due to micro-organisms are peculiarly adapted to prevention and control. This is due largely to the fact that before infection can occur the organisms must not only be present in the community but must be able to leave the source where they have been multiplying, they must travel some distance in the outside world from the source to the patient, and the patient himself must be susceptible to infection. It is, therefore, possible to break this chain of causation at each of these three points, by controlling the sources of pathogenic micro-organisms, by cutting their lines of communication or by rendering the population refractory to infection. The techniques required for these purposes will be discussed in this and the succeeding three chapters.

Except for tetanus and gas gangrene, whose source is the soil, all the remaining pathogens come from human beings or the animal kingdom. Preventing infection by dealing with its source will, therefore, involve some form of control of animals or human beings whom we suspect may be infected by, or who are carriers of pathogenic organisms. Several methods are available for this purpose.

Procedures at ports and frontiers

Some forms of infection do not occur in many countries for the simple reason that the causative organisms are not there. If, therefore, they can be kept out, freedom from these diseases will obviously continue.

It is by this method that Great Britain has been kept free from rabies because the importation of all dogs has been prohibited for many years and it is only after it has been kept-in strict quarantine for six months to make certain that it is not in the incubation stage of the disease that one is allowed to enter.

Human beings may likewise be in the incubation stage or actually suffering from diseases that are unknown in this country. For this reason, every ship coming to Britain for example, from ports outside Europe is boarded on arrival by Port Medical Officers who ascertain what illnesses have occurred on the voyage, and may even inspect passengers and crew if they suspect that anyone is suffering from such a disease as cholera or plague. Not until the Medical Officer is satisfied that they are free from infections that are unknown here, is the ship given a clean bill of health and landing is permitted.

Passengers who arrive by air cannot be controlled quite so easily but they too may be in the incubation stage of diseases such as cholera. They are accordingly warned that they must report any illness they may contract during the 14 days after arrival. In addition, many countries also require that incoming passengers shall have been immunized against such diseases as cholera, and yellow fever.

Procedures within the country

When the micro-organism responsible for a disease is already in the country, little is to be gained from control measures to prevent its importation. But it may be possible to confine the organism and keep it away from the general population, if patients in the acute stage of the disease or apparently normal persons known to be carriers can be suitably controlled.

It is for this reason that many infectious diseases must be reported to the local Health Authority within 48 hours of their diagnosis. In Great Britain, they comprise the following:-

1. *Diseases which are primarily infections of the respiratory*

tract or due to organisms known to be derived from the respiratory tract.

Diphtheria, scarlet fever, acute meningitis, tuberculosis, whooping cough and measles.

2. *Diseases which are primarily infections of the intestinal tract and in which the organisms are present in the faeces of patients or carriers.*

Cholera, enteric fever (typhoid and paratyphoid fever), dysentery, poliomyelitis and food infection.

3. *Diseases connected with childbirth.*

Ophthalmia neonatorum.

4. *Animal diseases transmissible to man.*

Anthrax, brucellosis, leptospirosis and plague.

5. *Others not included in the above.*

Hepatitis, typhus, acute encephalitis, tetanus, yellow fever, malaria, Lassa fever, leprosy, Marburg disease and viral haemorrhagic fever.

When patients with these diseases are notified, it is the duty of the appropriate Officer of the Local Health Authority to ensure that the patient is not only properly treated but is cared for in such a way that he is not likely to become a danger to others. The actual procedure employed varies according to circumstances, but generally involves some form of isolation of the patient and control of contacts or carriers.

Isolation in hospitals

For many reasons, the most satisfactory method is to send the patient to an isolation ward or hospital. After his departure, the bedroom should be fumigated with formaldehyde gas, the mattress and bedding autoclaved and library books destroyed. These matters are usually attended to by the Environment Health Officer.

But the matter does not end at this point. The family should be kept under observation so that further cases can be dealt with promptly. Any children in the household should be kept from school. As a general rule, adults can go to work, but if this involves the preparation or handling of food and the patient has had an infection of the intestinal tract, they too should remain at home. If the disease involved is diphtheria, all contacts should be immunized.

Barrier nursing

In some forms of infection, particularly typhoid and para-typhoid fevers and tuberculosis, the diagnosis may not be made until the patient has already been in hospital for some time and for various reasons it may be inadvisable to move him to an isolation hospital or sanatorium. In such instances the patient should be transferred to a single room failing which the only recourse is the procedure known as *barrier nursing*.

This is difficult and should be avoided if possible. It entails retaining the patient in the same ward as other patients but employing procedures designed to protect the latter against infection by his organisms. His bed, for example, should be placed at one end of the ward and near a wash basin. Screens, preferably made of plastic, should be placed round the bed and kept there until he is discharged.

The rest of the technique can only be mastered as a result of practical experience but it involves the wearing of gowns and masks by everyone entering the screened area, and the use of disposable china and cutlery. Great care is also taken with everything coming out of the screened area to ensure that pathogenic organisms are not conveyed to others. Bedclothes should, therefore be placed in an impervious bag that can be sealed completely. Stools and urine must also be rendered harmless by treatment with a strong antiseptic.

Immediately after attending such patients, the nurse must wash her hands, if possible, in a separate bowl. If this cannot be arranged, she must rinse her hands in antiseptic before using a communal bowl. Disposable paper towels must be used whenever possible.

Control of carriers

In the preceding sections only frank cases of infection or patients in the incubation stage of disease were considered. But in many forms of infection, carriers are equally important as sources of the organisms. Although they should, theoretically, be treated in the same way as patients with the disease this is seldom possible.

This is partly due to the fact that they can only be detected as a result of bacteriological examination and partly because an individual who feels perfectly well does not submit kindly to interference with his liberty. Nevertheless, great care should be taken that a patient recovered from diphtheria, typhoid or paratyphoid is kept under some form of supervision if he is known to be a convalescent carrier of the organism concerned. This may necessitate repeated bacteriological examination of the throat or stools. Attempts to prevent spread of other diseases by detection of individuals who may be convalescent carriers are not usually made.

Carriers may also be detected when search is being made for the probable sources of the organisms causing epidemics. This generally occurs with typhoid or paratyphoid fever and when discovered the individual is usually found to be a permanent carrier who has either had the disease many years ago or has become a carrier for no known reason. Although such individuals can be prohibited from working in restaurants, etc., and be warned to wash their hands after defaecation, there is little else that can be done with them. Attempts to rid them of their organisms are not always successful.

Attempts are sometimes made to prevent carriers of certain organisms from having too close contact with particularly vulnerable members of the population. It is for this reason a common practice to ascertain whether the staffs of maternity departments are carriers of pathogenic streptococci and to exclude them until they are free. Carriers of staphylococci are generally too numerous to be sent off duty.

Respiratory infections
Intestinal infections
Infection of wounds
Gas gangrene and
  tetanus

Staphylococcal infection
  in nurseries
Puerperal infections
Insect-borne infections

5

Prevention of infection by cutting the lines of communication

In many forms of infection it is impracticable to isolate all cases of the disease or to find and deal suitably with the carriers. Nevertheless, the organisms from both cases and carriers may be kept from susceptible individuals by various methods, all of which involve cutting the lines of communication by which the organisms travel. The methods employed—and the success achieved—depend to a very large extent on the type of infection involved.

Respiratory infections

Except for diphtheria and whooping cough which can be prevented by previous immunization of susceptible members of the community, very little has so far been achieved in preventing infections of the respiratory tract by inhibiting the passage of the organisms from person to person. It is for this reason that such common infections as colds and influenza are still virtually uncontrolled. Tuberculosis is, however, an exception in that the tubercule bacilli in his sputum can be prevented from reaching others if the patient is kept in hospital until they have ceased to be expectorated. If circumstances are such that this is not possible, he should at least be taught to expectorate into a suitably covered receptacle and invariably to use disposable handkerchiefs.

Intestinal infections

Except for cases of intestinal infection due to the consumption of meat or meat products from infected animals, the great majority are due to the presence in food or drink of organisms which have come from the faeces of cases or carriers. It therefore follows that much may be done to prevent these infections if, firstly, the excreta are disposed of in such a way that any pathogens they contain cannot reach others and, secondly all food and drink consumed by the community is guarded against contamination at its source or while in transit to the consumer.

Measures designed to effect this have now been employed in all civilized countries for many years and it is in consequence of this that many forms of intestinal infection have either disappeared entirely or have become very unusual. This particularly applies to cholera, typhoid, paratyphoid and the more severe varieties of dysentery, all of which were at one time common but have now become very unusual in Northern Europe and North America. Further details of the techniques required are given below.

Disposal of excreta

The most efficient method for the disposal of excreta is by the water carriage system in which it is carried in a stream of water to sewage disposal plants where pathogenic organisms are destroyed by the action of other species of bacteria before the sewage is allowed to discharge into a water-course or the sea. When it is not possible to provide such a system it is necessary to have recourse to chemical closets, cesspits, latrines, privies or buckets. With all of these, there is much more danger that faecal organisms may reach others but a great deal can be done to prevent this if earth or sand is used to cover the excreta, flies are prevented from reaching it, and the containers are emptied frequently, their contents being buried in soil where they can remain until decomposition is complete.

Whatever method be ultimately employed for the disposal of faeces and urine, the napkins and bedpans that must be used by infants and patients who are confined to bed, are a source of real danger to others. For pathogenic organisms in them can reach others in a variety of ways. Prevention of this is a direct responsibility of the nurse.

The methods that should be used for their treatment are described in more detail on pages 116 and 119 but it should be mentioned at this point that if disposable napkins, which are the ideal, cannot be used, the treatment of the cotton squares that are the only alternative, should take place somewhere distant from the nursery and by personnel who have nothing to do with the preparation of feeds for the babies.

Control of food and drink

Food that is eaten immediately after cooking is not likely to contain pathogenic organisms because the temperature reached is usually sufficient to kill them. But when the food is eaten without cooking as is the case with fruit or the ingredients of salads, or alternatively is not eaten until it has been kept for some time after cooking, organisms of all kinds, and particularly faecal organisms, can reach it in a variety of ways described in more detail on page 58. Much however can be done to prevent contamination by keeping prepared foods as far away as possible from raw foods combined with strict attention to cleanliness in the kitchen and the use of water with a temperature of 80°C (176°F) for washing up. This temperature is usually adequate to kill pathogens. Contamination of the food by flies can be prevented by insecticides, screening of windows and muslin or wire mesh covers for exposed foods. Transfer of faecal organisms on the hands of the cook can be prevented by requiring that the hands be washed after defaecation.

Milk may also contain pathogenic organisms. It is partly for this reason that nearly all the milk consumed in large cities has been pasteurized, that is, held at a temperature of 63–65°C (145–149°F) for thirty minutes. And if this process has been properly carried out there is no doubt that such milk is not likely to contain organisms capable of causing disease. If the milk has not been pasteurized it should be brought to the boil

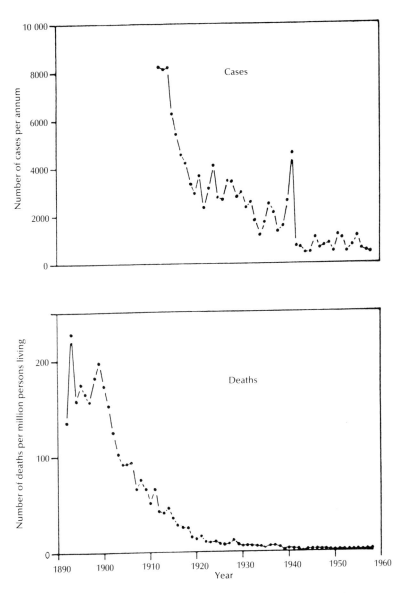

Fig. 5.1 Disappearance of typhoid and paratyphoid fevers following the widespread introduction of the water-carriage system of sewage disposal, filtration, and chlorination of water supplies, pasteurization of milk, and similar measures.

and cooled as quickly as possible. Dried milk may also contain pathogenic organisms so that after it has been dissolved—preferably in boiled water—it should also be brought to the boil. Whenever possible all milk should be stored in a refrigerator in order to prevent growth of organisms, for it must never be forgotten that milk is an excellent culture medium.

When the milk is required for infants and young children, in hospital there is much to be said for commercially prepared bottled feeds. But if the milk feeds are to be prepared locally two methods are available. The first is to make up the feeds in clean bottles which are then either sterilized by autoclaving or pasteurized by immersion in a tank of water for 30 minutes at a temperature of 63–65°C (145–149°F). The second method involves preliminary disinfection of the bottles and teats by immersion in a chlorine containing antiseptic such as Milton for 2 hours and then filling with the feeds prepared under as clean conditions as possible.

Water is much less likely to contain faecal organisms than is food or milk. This is particularly the case if it comes from a municipal water supply because it has generally been treated in such a way as to kill or remove them. Filtration through sand and the addition of chlorine are usually employed for this purpose. But if it must be taken from a river, stream or shallow well without such treatment it may be necessary to boil it or add sufficient hypochlorous acid or other chlorine-containing compound to give a concentration of about 5 parts chlorine per million of water. Sets containing the necessary materials and apparatus and chemicals for ensuring that sufficient chlorine is present can be obtained in some countries. Addition of sufficient potassium permanganate (20 parts per million) to give the water a marked pink colour is an alternative method, but its efficiency is far below that of chlorine.

Infection of wounds

Before the discovery by Lord Lister, that infection of wounds was due to micro-organisms, no precautions whatever were taken to prevent them reaching wounds. In consequence, every wound of any size inevitably became infected. Serious at any time, this was at its worst in hospitals where cross infection of operation wounds as well as those due to trauma was responsible for an appallingly high incidence of gas gangrene and tetanus as well as pyogenic infection. The introduction of asepsis into surgical procedures was followed by the virtual disappearance of tetanus and gas gangrene and a very considerable reduction in the incidence of pyogenic infection. But aseptic methods will not alone prevent wound infection. Much else is required, and it is for this reason that infection of wounds is still comparatively common.

A great deal can, however, be done, but for several reasons it is advisable to consider traumatic wounds separately from those resulting from clean operations.

Traumatic wounds

These may have the spores of the tetanus and gas gangrene bacilli in them at the time of infliction. Staphylococci may also be present but are more likely to reach them some time afterwards. This also applies to streptococci, Pseudomonas and coliform bacilli.

Every effort must be made when the wound is first seen to clean it as much as possible, removing all foreign bodies, and if there has been much destruction of tissue, anything that is dead or likely to die should also be dealt with. Whether antiseptics should be employed is extremely doubtful for reasons given on page 140.

At this dressing and indeed at all subsequent dressings the nurse must be conscious of the fact that she herself may be a carrier of staphylococci or streptococci and even if the wound appears to be dirty, it is quite possible that these organisms may have not yet reached it. She must, therefore, do nothing that will facilitate the transfer of her own organisms to the wound. Largely because her hands may be contaminated by organisms from her own throat or nose it follows that under no circumstances must the bare hands come into contact with the wound, the skin in its neighbourhood or the dressings. If it is necessary to use the hands for exploration, to insert stitches or palpate the wound or skin, gloves should invariably be worn. If sterile gloves are available so much the better but if not, pathogens will be removed from unsterilized gloves if they are put on and then washed thoroughly with soap and water.

It is also a common practice to wear masks, the theory being that they prevent infected droplets from the nose or mouth reaching the wound. There is no harm in this practice, but it is doubtful whether it is worth the trouble, for it is now known that the droplets only seldom contain the organisms that cause infection of wounds. In any event, droplets are not produced unless the carrier speaks, coughs or sneezes. Anyone with a cough or who has a cold so that he has to sneeze should not be dressing a wound at all; and speaking is not usually necessary when carrying out dressings. For these reasons, masks have little to recommend them.

Dressing technique. For most wounds, a method of dressing known as the 'no touch' (or 'non-touch') technique is the method of choice. The full details of this method of dressing wounds are adequately described in text-books and in any event can only be learnt by practice. Suffice it to say that care is taken before the operation starts, to have everything that is likely to be required, available in suitable receptacles on the trolley; that the hands of the dresser are then washed and dried on a sterile towel; and that neither the dressings nor the wound are touched by the hands, forceps being used for the entire operation except the removal and replacement of the bandages or binders.

One of the most important aspects of the whole technique is the disposal of the instruments and dirty dressings for if the wound is infected, they may be loaded with organisms. The dressings should, whenever possible, be placed direct into a disposable bag with as little agitation as possible, the bag closed and placed in a bin in the sluice room in which it must stay until the contents can be burnt.

Any disposable instruments should be included in the same bag as the dressings but those that must be used again should be placed in another bag which can be sealed and in which they are returned to the C.S.S.D. where they can be dealt with properly before use again. If there is no C.S.S.D., they must be made safe as soon as possible by thorough cleaning, followed by boiling or autoclaving before use again.

A second, and equally important point is that nurses who have some form of superficial infection such as furunculosis, a boil, stye or paronychia should not dress wounds and preferably should remain off duty until the infection is over.

Ward procedures. In view of the fact that cross infection may occur in wards even when the technique employed for dressing wounds is above reproach, a number of additional precautions should be taken whenever possible.

Removal of all infected patients to isolation wards should, if possible, be the rule. Unfortunately many hospitals do not possess such facilities; but barrier nursing is not an altogether suitable alternative partly because it has yet to be proved to be of value and partly because of the extra load thrown on the nursing staff.

Much may, however, be done by attempting to keep the number of infected particles in the air as small as possible and particularly during the period devoted to dressings. The best way to achieve this is the provision of a special dressing room where dressings can be carried out away from the airborne organisms that are inevitably present in the air of any surgical ward. Contamination of the air of the room itself by organisms reaching it from infected wounds while they are being dressed, can be prevented by installing forced-draught ventilation.

If such a room cannot be provided and dressings must be carried out in the ward itself, it is possible to keep the number of airborne organisms low by various methods. If possible, dust should be disposed of by a vacuum cleaner, impregnated mop or wet duster and certainly not by sweeping with a broom. Bedmaking should have been completed at least half and preferably a full hour before dressings are started.

Direct transfer of infection by instruments, dressings, etc., can be prevented by the sterilization procedures usually employed and the use of the no-touch technique when actually doing the dressings. But it is not unusual for surgeons and nurses who invariably employ the no-touch technique when dressing a wound, to use their bare hands to remove the dressings when they merely wish to inspect a wound. Indeed they may even go so far as actually to palpate the skin in the neighbourhood of the wound. This is a most dangerous proceeding which should be discouraged whenever possible because of the possibility that the individual may be a carrier. For this reason gloves must invariably be worn on such occasions. They need not have been sterilized, all that is necessary is to put them on and wash them thoroughly with soap under a running tap. It is not even essential to dry them, but if desired a sterile towel must of course be used. When a series of patients are being examined, the washing process must of course be repeated after each patient.

Transfer of organisms from patient to patient as a result of contamination of mattresses, blankets, pillows and the communal bath may be difficult to prevent but much may be done by the use of plastic covers for mattresses and pillows that can be wiped down with antiseptic, cotton blankets that can be boiled and the treatment of the bath with strong antiseptic every time it is used.

Clean operation wounds

As many as possible of the patient's own organisms should be removed before the operation starts by bathing, shaving and putting on clean clothing. The site of the operation is generally swabbed with antiseptic before the operation starts. Introduction of pathogens into the wound on instruments, swabs, dressing and towels can be prevented by adequate sterilization (see Ch. 6).

Transfer of organisms from carriers in the operating team can be minimized by washing their hands thoroughly, donning clean clothes before the operation and wearing gowns, caps, gloves and masks during the operation itself. Taking showers, frequently recommended in the past, has now been found to increase rather than decrease the dissemination of skin organisms during the operation and is best avoided. Every care must also be taken to minimize traffic into and outside the theatre while movement within the theatre should be kept to a minimum.

The precautions necessary to prevent the entry of pathogenic organisms into the wound after the operation are exactly the same as those outlined for traumatic wounds. But another series of precautions are necessary in genito-urinary wards because of the ability of the organisms that cause urinary infections to multiply in urine and so contaminate urinals and drainage bottles. Whenever possible, disposable urinals or sterile plastic bags should be employed. But if they are not available, and ordinary glass or metal urinals are the only alternative, they should certainly be sterilized after use by autoclaving or immersion in a strong antiseptic solution.

Gas gangrene and tetanus

The probable sources of the organisms and the way in which they reach wounds have already been discussed in Chapter 3. And since the spores may be present in dust, dirt and faeces, it follows that they may enter traumatic wounds at the time of infliction. It is for this reason that children should, whenever possible be immunized with tetanus toxoid. It is also advisable for adults and particularly those, such as farmers and builders who come into contact with the sources of these organisms (see Ch. 7). It is, unfortunately not yet possible to obtain protection against gas gangrene in this way.

Much may also be done to prevent these diseases if, following infliction of the wound, it is thoroughly cleansed with debridement if necessary.

Infections of this nature are very unusual after clean operations but the fact that they can occur and that the spores of the organisms concerned have been found on the shelves, ledges and floors of operating theatres, emphasizes the importance of extreme cleanliness not only in operating theatres, but in casualty and out-patient departments where any form of operative interference is carried out.

If, despite these precautions, tetanus or gas gangrene occur, the technique outlined under Infection of Wounds above is, in general, adequate to prevent transfer of organisms to other patients.

Staphylococcal infection in nurseries

When staphylococci produce infection in new-born babies they may have come from one or other of four sources; (1) other babies with some form of clinically obvious infection; (2) nurses who have some trivial infection; (3) babies whose umbilicus is supporting the growth of staphylococci without showing signs of infection, and (4) nurses who are carriers.

The first two of these sources should, if possible, be removed from the nursery forthwith. The third source can be rendered less dangerous if the umbilicus is dressed in such a way that its organisms cannot reach the fingers or clothing of anyone who attends to it.

This leaves the fourth source, the nurse who is a carrier, to be dealt with. Since it is undoubtedly the organisms on her fingers and clothing that actually reach the baby, she should attend to the baby in such a way that it does not come into contact with her ordinary clothes. The best method is to carry out this operation on a table, but if this is not available and the baby must be placed on the nurse's lap, she should wear a plastic waterproof apron which can be wiped down with an antiseptic. Her hands too must be carefully washed not only at the start of her activities in the nursery but between each baby. They must, moreover, be dried in some form of disposable towel, never on a communal roller towel. Since continual washing—particularly if it be properly carried out—is not good for the skin, treatment with an antiseptic cream containing Hibitane 1/1000 has been advocated.

Better still are gloves. If sterile disposable gloves are available they should be used. But even ordinary rubber gloves are better than nothing for all pathogenic organisms will be removed if they are washed with soap and water.

Puerperal infections

As long ago as 1846, the Hungarian obstetrician Semmelweis, found that many cases of puerperal fever or infection of the uterus after delivery could be prevented, if the hands of the obstetrician were carefully washed and treated with water containing chlorine before examining or handling the patient. As a result the incidence of the disease fell considerably.

Since then, a great deal has been learned about this disease and many other improvements in technique have been introduced.

As already mentioned in Chapter 3, infection of the uterus after delivery may be due to haemolytic streptococci derived from the throat of an attendant at delivery or anaerobic streptococci from the mother's own birth canal.

Prevention of the former type of infection necessitates employing sterile towels, gowns and instruments at the confinement. In fact the labour ward should be looked upon in very much the same way as an operating theatre and delivery carried out with the same ritual. If delivery takes place at home, there is no particular reason why the conditions should not approximate to those achieved in hospital. But wherever delivery takes place, it is the hands of the midwife or obstetrician to which most attention should be given for there seems little doubt that it is by way of the fingers contaminated from the midwife's own throat that infection occurs. For this reason, gloves must be worn.

Prevention of anaerobic streptococcal infections is best achieved by avoidance of any form of intra-uterine manipulation during or after delivery. Much may be done in this direction by adequate antenatal supervision.

Insect-borne infections

In many tropical countries the organisms causing infections such as yellow fever, dengue, typhus and relapsing fever are conveyed from person to person by insect vectors such as mosquitoes, lice and fleas. Control of these diseases usually involves measures for the eradication of these insects.

Mosquitoes are the vectors of yellow fever, dengue and encephalitis. It is generally necessary to ascertain the species responsible and find out its breeding habits because, on the whole, it is during the larval stage of the development of mosquitoes that they are most vulnerable. For, whatever the species, the larvae must live in water such as that of marshes, ponds or even slowly flowing rivers and streams. In the water they remain close to the surface in order to breathe. It is, therefore, possible to eradicate mosquitoes by draining the water; by suffocating the larvae as a result of spraying oil on the surface of the water; or by adding a poisonous chemical such as arsenic to the water itself.

In addition to these measures, screening of the windows and doors of dwelling houses to prevent entry of the mosquitoes that do succeed in hatching, together with mosquito nets for beds and the application of an insecticide in the houses, may do much to prevent the spread of these diseases. Indeed, yellow fever was completely eradicated from the Panama Canal Zone by measures of this description.

Louse-borne diseases such as typhus and relapsing fever require completely different measures because the louse lives on the hair and clothing of human beings. Eradication of lice by cutting short the hair, boiling, heating or steaming the clothing can only be successful if the individual can succeed in remaining clear of lice thereafter. Not only may this be very difficult but the measures themselves are too cumbersome to apply on a large scale. A more recent and much better method of eradication is by dusting with insecticides. But it must be borne in mind that insects can become resistant to these.

Flea-borne diseases, that is plague and one form of typhus, usually come from rats and in such instances the rats rather than the fleas are best attacked, but insecticide spraying of the floors of houses may also do much to prevent the disease.

6

Prevention of infection by sterilization and disinfection

In the preceding chapter the methods by which living organisms from patients or carriers can be prevented from reaching susceptible human beings did not, as a rule, involve killing the organisms. It is, however, possible to prevent some forms of infection by measures that result in their destruction before they reach the patient.

Two procedures can be employed for this purpose. One requires killing all the organisms and their spores and taking the necessary steps to prevent their return. This is usually described as *sterilization*. There are, however, many situations in medicine where this is either unnecessary or impossible but infection can still be prevented if *disinfection* is employed. This involves the destruction or elimination of any pathogens present at the time but, except for what can be achieved by cleanliness, taking no specific steps to prevent their return.

Many techniques are now available for this purpose, but it is of great importance that due regard be paid to their limitations for, under certain circumstances, nearly all of them may fail to achieve complete sterilization. This is largely due to the fact that micro-organisms vary considerably in their resistance to the procedures that are usually employed. Thus *vegetative organisms*, that is to say, cocci, bacilli, vibrios, spirochaetes and fungi, can be killed with comparative ease. So too can the *rickettsiae* and *viruses* but even so, some of the antiseptics that can kill vegetative organisms may have little, if any, effect on viruses. *Spores* (see p. 6) are the most resistant of all. They are very much more difficult to kill than any of the vegetative organisms, rickettsiae or viruses. So much so that it is largely because of their possible presence that many of the sterilizing procedures employed must be much more drastic than would be necessary to kill vegetative organisms and viruses.

Because of these complications, it is first necessary to discuss, in general terms, the different methods that can be employed to kill micro-organisms. With this as a basis, it will be possible to consider which of the available techniques is best suited for use in each of the many situations in medical practice where sterilization and disinfection are required.

METHODS EMPLOYED FOR STERILIZATION

Micro-organisms and their spores can be killed by both physical and chemical agents.

Physical agents

The physical agents that can kill micro-organisms are radiations and high temperatures.

Radiations

Many forms of radiation such as sunlight, X-rays, gamma rays, ultra-violet light and infra-red rays can kill micro-organisms.

Perhaps the most useful is gamma radiation. These are penetrating rays from a source of atomic energy such as radioactive cobalt. They will pass through almost anything except thick lead shields. They possess three advantages. They can sterilize articles that are already packed in sealed containers. Secondly, heat is not required so that articles that would be damaged by high temperatures can be easily sterilized. And, thirdly, the articles do not get wet, one of the disadvantages of sterilization by antiseptics.

This method possesses two main disadvantages. The first is the size and high cost of the apparatus, so that it is only when very large quantities can be dealt with that this method is feasible. The second is that there remain many parts of the world where distance, economic conditions and similar factors render its employment impossible or very difficult.

Nevertheless, it is by this method that most of the many disposable articles in sealed paper or plastic coverings now employed in medicine have been sterilized. It is unnecessary to describe the procedures employed by the manufacturers but the nurse must take certain precautions when using such articles.

1. If there is choice, only articles that have been packed in such a manner that they will not become contaminated while being withdrawn from the package should be employed. Such contamination can easily occur if there is only a single wrapper, since organisms on the outer surface may get on to the article while it is being withdrawn. To prevent this, two wrappers should be provided, the outer being completely sealed while the inner should not. This wrapper protects the article against contamination while it and the article within are being removed from the outer wrapper.
2. No article whose outer wrapper has been damaged should be used.
3. Once the wrapper is opened, the article must be used without delay.
4. The article must be destroyed after use.

High temperatures

Until quite recently, almost all the procedures employed for medical purposes depended on the fact that high temperatures can kill micro-organisms. But the introduction of instruments which are sterilized by radiation has rendered sterilization by heat a less common procedure. Nevertheless, the fact remains that there are many situations in medicine where sterilization by some form of heating must still be employed because of its simplicity, economy and applicability in almost any situation. Because of this the nurse may be forced to employ such methods and should know something about the correct procedures.

In whatever way the heat be applied, it is a matter of some

importance that the temperature required to effect complete sterilization and the time that will be necessary, depend to a very large extent on the presence or absence of water. For, in general, micro-organisms are killed much more easily in water or steam than by dry heat.

Dry heat

Dry air heated to a sufficiently high temperature can kill micro-organisms but quite long heating may be required. Staphylococci, for example, may be still alive after exposure for several hours to temperatures as high as 100°C (212°F). Spores, such as those of tetanus and gas gangrene bacilli, are also unaffected at this temperatures. At higher temperatures such as 120°C (248°F), staphylococci are soon killed but spores may survive. Indeed, it is not until the temperature reaches 150°C (302°F) that those of tetanus bacilli are killed. Even so, it may take as long as 30 minutes. At still higher temperatures, shorter times will suffice, so that 12 minutes at 160°C (320°F), 5 minutes at 170°C (338°F) and only one minute at 180°C (356°F) will kill all the tetanus spores exposed to these temperatures.

In practice, a temperature of 160°C is usually employed, maintained for one hour to provide a sufficient margin of safety. Needless to say, so high a temperature can seriously damage cloth, rubber and plastics. Because of this, hot air should only be used for the sterilization of glass or metallic articles such as syringes, needles and knives. A further drawback is that if the method is to be entirely safe a specially built oven is essential to provide an even temperature at all levels. For these reasons, hot air is only seldom employed at the present time.

Moist heat

When the heat is conveyed to the organisms in water or steam, it is possible to kill them at lower temperatures and in shorter times than when dry hot air is used. This difference is due to the fact that the organisms are killed as a result of entirely different processes. When water is present, no matter whether it is liquid or in the form of steam, death of the organisms is due to coagulation of their proteins. When water is not present, coagulation does not occur until very high temperatures indeed are reached. Long before this, the heat has brought about oxidation and it is this which kills the organisms. Nevertheless the temperature required to bring about oxidation is always higher than that required to cause coagulation of the proteins.

Table 6.1 Time required for complete sterilization of tubercle bacilli in milk

Temperature (°C)	Time necessary to kill all tubercle bacilli
55.6	60 min
57.8	30 min
60.0	15 min
65.6	2 min
71.1	30 sec
76.7	20 sec

Water. The great majority of the vegetative organisms and viruses are killed after immersion for only a few minutes in water at as low a temperature as 60°C (140°F). Some such as the tubercle bacillus may require exposure for as long as 15 minutes and other species more than 30 minutes (see Table 6.1). But when the temperature is raised to that of boiling water 100°C (212°F), all these organisms are killed in a few seconds.

Spores are much more likely to be resistant. Virtually none are killed in water at 60°C (140°F). At 100°C (212°F), the great majority are killed within a minute but those of some species may require 10 to 15 minutes. Indeed, the spores of some strains of tetanus and gas gangrene bacilli have been known to survive boiling for several hours.

It has, however, been found that such highly resistant spores are very unusual indeed. Articles that are scrupulously clean and free of dust, dirt or soil are certainly not likely to be contaminated by such spores. In practice, therefore, it has been found that instruments, etc., that have been boiled in water for only 3–5 minutes are sterile—all bateria, fungi, viruses and spores having been killed.

It is for this reason that boiling water can generally quite safely be employed in medical practice to render such objects as instruments, syringes, porringers and bowls free of all living micro-organisms. We therefore refer to them as 'sterile' and the containers in which they have been boiled as 'sterilizers'.

Nevertheless, the fact remains that if, by chance, the articles submitted to this operation were contaminated by unusually resistant spores, they might survive and the articles would, in fact, not be sterile. It is for this reason that it is now accepted practice in developed countries for articles to be sterilised by autoclaving or by some other process that can be relied upon to kill spores.

Partly because so many articles that were previously sterilized by boiling have now become available from central sterilizing departments or commercial sources, sterilization by boiling water is not only looked upon with disfavour nowadays but nurses may not even be taught how to do it or the precautions that must be taken to ensure its success. Nevertheless, there are still many parts of the world where boiling in water may be the only method available. It is accordingly advisable to give further details.

The water may be contained in a vessel of almost any size or shape as long as it is deep enough to ensure that the articles are covered and the water is actually boiling. A rectangular container with a hinged counter-balanced lid and heated by gas, electricity or steam is useful. The lid should fit properly so that steam does not emerge in excessive amounts. The water must be boiling and to ensure this the best models possess a thermometer. On the other hand it must not boil so furiously that the water level quickly falls because of evaporation. A tray, which can be lifted clear of the water, should from part of the equipment so that the instruments can be quickly removed from the depths of the sterilizer without it being necessary to fish for them with forceps. When the water is hard, calcium salts come out of solution during the boiling and may be deposited on the instruments or, in the form of scale, on the sides of the instrument itself. Periodical cleaning is, therefore, imperative.

But perhaps the most important points of all are that the articles must be totally immersed and that boiling must continue for at least 3 and preferably 5 minutes. To ensure this an egg timer may be used and if it is placed on the lid of the sterilizer, there will be no temptation to remove the instruments prematurely.

When the boiling period is over, the articles can be removed by Cheatle's forceps and placed direct into a sterilized kidney dish or similar receptacle. Since they will be hot, they must be allowed to cool before being used. This process may take a little time and airborne organisms may reach them. For this reason, they should be covered by a sterile towel until needed.

Water is also employed in the process known as *pasteurization* which entails immersion of the articles in water at a temperature of 70–80°C (176–194°F) for 30 minutes. Although this cannot sterilize them in the usual sense of the term, it can kill the pathogenic organisms likely to be present on them. This method is generally employed for articles that would be damaged by boiling water or steam. Milk is also treated by pasteurization but the temperature employed may be lower, only 63–65°C (145–149°F).

Steam. Steam is a much more efficient sterilizing agent than water boiling in an open vessel. One reason for this is that the temperature can be very much higher. The highest temperature that water or steam can reach when boiling in a kettle or saucepan is 100°C (212°F). This is at sea level and it may be very much lower in countries such as Ethiopia or Mexico whose altitude may approach 3,000 metres. But if it is boiled in a completely closed vessel so that the steam cannot escape, very much higher temperatures can be obtained.

The second reason for the greater efficiency of steam is that it contains latent heat, that is, the extra amount of heat that must be imparted to it to convert it from water into steam. This naturally adds to its value as a sterilizing agent. A third advantage of steam is that when properly used, the sterilized articles are dry at the end of the sterilizing process.

When exposed to steam at 100°C (212°F), all the vegetative organisms and viruses are killed within a few seconds. Spores may survive for longer periods. Those of some of the gas gangrene bacilli for example, are not killed until they have been in steam at 100°C (212°F) for as long as 10 minutes. At 115°C (239°F), only 5 minutes are required and at 120°C (248°F), one minute will suffice. It is thus obvious that steam is one of the most efficient sterilizing agents we possess.

Because the steam must be under pressure if it is to reach a sufficiently high temperature, it is necessary to employ a vessel that can be closed tightly enough to prevent escape of the steam. This vessel is usually known as an *autoclave*. The simplest of all is the ordinary domestic pressure cooker in which

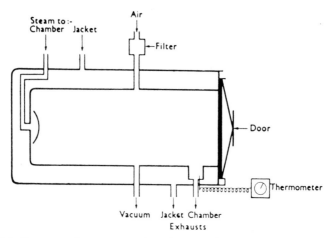

Fig. 6.1 Diagrammatic representation of an autoclave.

the steam is generated from water inside the vessel by placing it over a suitable source of heat such as a gas ring, electric hot plate or primus stove.

More satisfactory is a larger cylindrical vessel such as that illustrated in Figure 6.1. The steam comes from a tank placed underneath heated by whatever means may be most convenient. Larger vessels generally supplied with steam from the hospital boilers may sometimes be available.

But whatever their size these autoclaves are fundamentally horizontal cylinders with a hinged door at one end. The shell of the autoclave is constructed in such a way that it is really two cylinders, one within the other, and enclosing a space or jacket into which steam can be admitted. This is provided so that the interior can be heated sufficiently to dry the articles after sterilization is completed.

Although autoclaves are usually operated by people specially trained for this purpose, it is by no means unusual in remote situations for nurses to have to do so or at least supervise their operation. For this reason they should know something about the process.

Operation of an autoclave. It is of the very greatest importance that whoever operates an autoclave must be aware that the agency that will sterilize the articles put into it is the steam, and not the air in the autoclave at the start which eventually becomes heated by the steam. It has already been stressed that steam at a temperature of 120°C is a most efficient sterilizing agent, whereas air at this temperature is singularly ineffective. It is therefore necessary to remove all the air from the auto-clave and from any containers put into it and replace the air by live steam.

Two methods are available for this. One is to remove the air by a vacuum pump and then admit steam which will fill the spaces from which the air came. The second is the so-called downward displacement method in which the air is actually pushed out of the autoclave. This is achieved by taking advantage of the fact that air is heavier than steam. In consequence, steam entering an autoclave tends to collect at its upper levels and the air at the lower. If therefore a valve is provided in the bottom of the autoclave and this is open, the air will drain out of the autoclave and be gradually replaced by steam. Not until all the air has been removed in this way, can the process of sterilization actually begin.

In whatever way the air has been removed from the auto-clave, the steam entering it will at first be at the same pressure as that of the atmosphere and at this pressure, its temperature can be only 100°C. But if all the valves and doors communicating with the outside are now closed, the pressure of steam

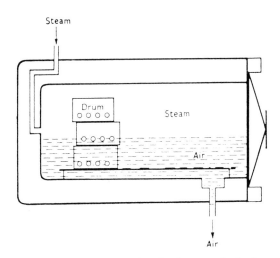

Fig. 6.2 Removal of air from an autoclave by downwards displacement.

will rise. At the same time, the temperature of the steam will also rise. There is close correlation between the pressure and the temperature so that when the pressure rises to 6 lb per square inch the temperature should be 110°C; at 10 lb it will be 115°C and at 15 lb 120°C and at 20 lb 125°C.

Unless special apparatus has been installed, more specifically referred to on page 107, it is usual to allow the pressure to increase to 15 or 20 lb per square inch and then close the steam valve sufficiently to prevent the pressure going higher. A safety valve arranged to blow off at this pressure may also be provided.

Once the desired pressure inside the chamber has been reached, it must be maintained for 30 minutes. Only 20 minutes sometimes suffices, but with large autoclaves and heavy loads the longer period is desirable. At the end of whatever period is employed, the valve in the steam inlet must be closed. The steam inside the chamber must now be removed. If not, it will condense and wet the articles. Its removal can be affected by allowing it to blow off into the open air through a pipe. A much better method is to use a pump not only to remove the steam but to produce a vacuum or partial vacuum in the chamber.

To assist in the drying process, the interior of the autoclave must be heated by allowing steam to circulate through the jacket. If these operations are carried out properly everything within should be completely dry within a few minutes.

Air must now be admitted to the chamber to enable the doors to be opened and the contents removed. Unfortunately, air contains an appreciable number of organisms so that unless it is filtered on its way into the autoclave they will contaminate the articles that have just been sterilized. The design of such filters and the substances used for filtration are both matters that have not yet reached finality. But there is no doubt that some form of air filtration is necessary, that it must be efficient and that it may require frequent attention to ensure its efficiency.

When the autoclave is once more full of air, it is then possible to open the door and remove the articles that have been sterilized.

Even so, the operation is not yet completely over because it is customary to remove the articles while they are still hot.

If they are to be used at once, as is the case with instruments on trays in theatre autoclaves this is of little importance. But many articles will not be used for some time and have usually been autoclaved in some form of container or covering. They will begin to cool at once and while doing so, the air inside the coverings will shrink so that air from the outside will be drawn into them to make up the difference. The amount of air that gets into them in this way is quite considerable being usually about a third of the volume of the container. Unfortunately, this air contains organisms so that the articles may have become contaminated soon after they have been sterilized.

This hazard can, to a large extent, be overcome by packing the articles in a suitable manner. Basically, this should consist of two separate coverings. The first consists of small parcels in paper or cloth wrappers generally referred to as *packs*, containing all the articles required for one precedure. A number of them are then placed in a *container* which is sufficiently porous to allow steam to penetrate into its interior but sufficiently robust to prevent organisms getting in while cooling or as a result of mechanical injury during transport and storage. Stout paper or cloth will suffice for this purpose but better still are cardboard boxes with deep fitting lids.

High vacuum, high temperature sterilization. Largely because the autoclaves described in the preceding section require up to 2 hours to complete the sterilization cycle, it is now becoming common practice to employ autoclaves whose cycle of operation lasts only 10–15 minutes. This can be achieved if a very powerful vacuum pump is employed that produces a complete vacuum in the chamber within 2–3 minutes. This is followed by steam at the unusually high temperature of 132°C which provides a pressure of about 30 pounds per square inch. Steam at this temperature and pressure sterilizes in only 2–3 minutes. The steam is then allowed to escape into the air and a complete vacuum once again produced. This should dry the articles within the autoclave some of which may have become wet as a result of condensation of the steam.

By using suitable apparatus, the operation of such an autoclave can be made entirely automatic. But such autoclaves are extremely expensive and only suitable for the sterilization of instruments in theatres or dressings in central sterile supply departments.

Low temperature steam sterilization. This method employs steam at a temperature of only 80–90°C and is used for the treatment of articles such as blankets, or rubber and plastic ware that would be harmed by higher temperatures. Its main disadvantage is that although vegetative forms of organisms are killed, spores may remain alive.

Low temperature steam and formalin vapour sterilization. If *formalin vapour is mixed with steam at a temperature of* 80–90°C the efficiency of the latter becomes much greater. So much so that spores may be killed. Although suitable for the sterilization of articles that might be harmed by higher temperatures, a specially adapted autoclave is required.

Tests for the efficiency of autoclaves. It is now common practice to carry out periodical checks that an autoclave is operating satisfactorily. One, perhaps the most important, is periodic inspeciton by an engineer to ascertain whether the correct internal temperature is being reached, that the vacuum pump removes all the air and that the timing mechanism is operating properly. A second is the incorporation of test objects in the loads going into the autoclave. Several are available. Browne's tubes are sealed glass tubes containing a chemical substance which turns from red to green if the required temperature has been reached in the autoclave. The second method is the so-called Bowie Dick technique. This comprises a pack of folded huckaback towels in the centre of which is a St Andrew's cross made of adhesive tape in which are incorporated strips of a chemical that is invisible before use but which becomes black if steam at the required temperature has reached them. A third method is the use of envelopes containing paper impregnated with bacterial spores. Unless they have been exposed to steam at the correct temperature, they will survive and grow if the paper is placed in a suitable culture medium.

There is no doubt that such tests are essential for the proper control of complex modern autoclaving procedures.

CHEMICAL AGENTS

In view of the fact that micro-organisms consist largely of protein, any chemical substance that can combine with protein will so injure the organisms that they will probably die. A great many chemical compounds such as strong acids and alkalis can act in this way, but cannot be employed for sterilization procedures in medicine because they might harm the objects which come into contact with them, and would certainly do great injury to patients if they reached wounds, skin or mucous membranes.

Many substances have, however, been evolved which do kill micro-organisms and have little deleterious effect on textiles, rubber, metals, etc., with which they come into contact. They are called *disinfectants* or *antiseptics*. There is a subtle distinction between the two terms in that a disinfectant is supposed to resemble a blunder-buss which kills every organism, whereas an antiseptic is considered to confine its activities to pathogenic organisms only. Since very few, if any, disinfectants or antiseptics behave as defined the distinction is artificial. Nor is it necessary and the term antiseptic only will be used in this book.

A great many antiseptics are now available. They vary greatly in their ability to kill micro-organisms, the time they will take to do so and how they will behave under the conditions in which they are called upon to act. These variations require a little more discussion.

Variations in susceptibility to antiseptics. It has already been mentioned that the spores produced by some species of bacteria such as the tetanus, gas gangrene and anthrax bacilli, are completely resistant to strong solutions of most antiseptics. Indeed, only somewhat unusual antiseptics such as formaldehyde in the form of gas or dissolved in water (formalin), glutaraldehyde and ethylene oxide gas can be depended upon to kill spores.

The vegetative forms of bacteria are, however, much more susceptible. With certain exceptions, referred to more specifically below, all are killed quickly and sometimes in high dilution by all the antiseptics referred to in Table 6.2.

One exception is the tubercle bacillus which is not killed by compounds that depend on chlorine for their activity.

A second and very important exception is *Pseudomonas*. This organism is so resistant that it can actually grow in the presence of cetrimide, in concentrations that kill other organisms.

Table 6.2 Compounds employed as antiseptics

Active principle	Compounds employed	Remarks
Halogens Iodine	Tincture of iodine Iodophors (Betadine)	Employed for skin sterilization
Chlorine	Chlorine gas	Used for drinking water
	Hypochlorous acid, Eusol, Dakin's solution Milton, Chloros, Deosan	Employed for wound irrigation Strong antiseptics. Valuable for viruses but no action on tubercle bacilli
Phenolics Phenols	Hycolin, Printol, Stericol	Strong general purposes antiseptics. Some viruses unaffected
Cresols	Lysol, Izal, Sudol, Cyllin, Ialine, Jeyes Fluid White fluid, Black fluid	Strong general purposes antiseptics. Little action on viruses. Corrosive in high concentration
Chloroxylenols	Dettol	Weaker antiseptics. Little action on *Pseudomonas*
Alcohols Ethyl alcohol Isopropyl alcohol	Industrial or surgical spirit	Very weak antiseptics. Used for skin preparation
Diguanides Chlorhexidine	Hibitane	Harmless in 1 per cent concentration. Valuable for staphylococci. No action on tubercle bacilli or viruses

Piclodoxine diglutonate	Resiguard	General purpose antiseptic
Aldehydes		
Glutaraldehyde	Cidex	Powerful antiseptic. Acts on both spores and viruses
Formaldehyde	Formalin gas	Employed for fumigation and sterilization with steam
	Formalin solution, Liq. formaldehyde B.P.C.	Very strong antiseptic but too irritating for general use
Quaternary ammonium compounds		
Cetyltrimethyl ammonium bromide	Cetavlon, Cetrimide	Used for skin and wounds. No action on tubercle bacilli or spores
Benzalkonium chloride	Zephiran, Roccal	
Surface active compounds		
Tego compounds		Skin disinfection and general purposes. No action on spores
Gas		
Ethylene oxide	Ethylene oxide mixed with an inert gas such as freon or carbon dioxide	Explosive and activity depends on humidity. Useful for apparatus

A third and even more important exception are the viruses. Many are unaffected by otherwise powerful antiseptics such as the phenols and cresols. On the other hand, they are highly susceptible to chlorine containing compounds.

Presence of other substances besides antiseptics. When proteins such as blood, serum, pus or faeces are present, they may seriously diminish the activity of antiseptics. The protein and antiseptic usually combine in such a way that the antiseptic is neutralized and ceases to act. For this reason, strong solutions must be employed.

Time required for an antiseptic to act. Antiseptics take an appreciable time to act. Experiments have shown that when staphylococci are smeared and dried on surfaces such as aluminium or rubber, immersion in a strong antiseptic such as phenol 1/20 will kill all the organisms in less than 30 seconds. But when subjected to the action of other antiseptics in the dilutions that are usually employed, considerably longer times may be required to kill the organisms. But provided the articles are made of a hard impenetrable substance such as metal, glass or porcelain, and that they are scrupulously clean, any antiseptic that can act at all should have done its work in 15 to 30 minutes. If however faeces, pus or other substances are present it may be advisable to allow anything from 2 to 12 hours. One thing is however quite certain, that merely dipping an instrument into an antiseptic in the hope of sterilizing it is asking too much.

The employment of antiseptics in medicine

Antiseptics have been and, indeed, are still used in medicine with two objectives in view. One is complete sterilization with no living organisms still present at the end of the process. The other is the killing of any pathogens that may be present without attempting to achieve complete sterility. Both must be discussed in a little more detail.

Complete sterilization. Because of their many deficiencies, antiseptics are of very limited value for this purpose and, on the whole, should only be used when there is no other alternative. They are accordingly employed for the treatment of plastic inserts, or optical and electrical apparatus that would be damaged by other methods of sterilization such as heat,

water or steam. Furthermore, only the more powerful compounds such as glutaraldehyde, ethylene oxide and formaldehyde should be used. Even so, each possess disadvantages.

Glutaraldehyde is employed as a solution in water and
although efficient when prepared, becomes valueless in a few
days.

Ethylene oxide is a gas that is so explosive that it must be
mixed with an inert gas before it can be used at all. An airtight
chamber is essential, several hours' exposure may be required
and its efficiency depends so much on the humidity and temperature that the method is best reserved for materials that
cannot be sterilized in any other way.

Formaldehyde can be employed as a solution in water or liberated from pellets in the form of a gas. Neither method is at
all satisfactory. The solution may damage many articles and the
gas may be unable to penetrate into close packed objects such
as piles of blankets or mattresses. It has however been found
that when incorporated in the steam employed in the low temperature method of steam sterilization described on page 108
the efficiency of the method is increased.

*Killing of pathogens but without attempting to achieve com-
plete sterility.* Antiseptics have been extensively employed for
this purpose. They include the treatment of discharges from
the body such as faeces, urine and pus or the containers into
which they have been deposited, that is to say, bed pans, napkins, and urinals. They are also used for the treatment of those
parts of the environment that such organisms are likely to have
reached, namely, walls, floors, sinks and baths. Bedding too
has occasionally been treated with them.

A third situation in which they are used is to kill pathogenic
organisms is on the hands of surgeons or the skin of the
patient through which an incision will be made. For much the
same reason, they are incorporated in the jellies and creams
used as lubricants during the insertion of catheters or vaginal
speculae.

A fourth use to which they are put is their inclusion in injection fluids such as vaccines or solutions for instillation into the
eye. But in this particular instance, all they are called upon to
do is to prevent growth of accidental contaminants.

Partly because it has been found that pathogens are much
less likely to be present than had previously been thought to

be the case in some situations such as on walls and even floors, and partly because of their unreliability, the employment of antiseptics in hospital practice is becoming less common. Other and much more efficient methods involving the use of heat in various forms are now supplanting them.

Nevertheless, if for various reasons, these methods cannot be employed and antiseptics are the only alternative, it is improbable that the nurse will be called upon to choose which one to use. It should be added that there is little connection between the cost of an antiseptic and its efficiency. Some of the most expensive have been evolved for use in certain situations where they are of sufficient value to justify their cost but are no better than many others when employed as general purpose antiseptics. Nor must it be forgotten that being commercially produced substances they are not exempt from the arts of sales promotion.

Whatever antiseptic is employed it is generally the nurse who will have to use it. So he or she must make certain that it is the correct antiseptic for the particular purpose in view, that its strength is adequate and that it has not been kept so long that it has deteriorated.

STERILIZATION AND DISINFECTION IN MEDICAL PRACTICE

For many years, the nurse was responsible for all the sterilization and disinfection required in hospital or private practice. But three developments have relieved her of much of this responsibility. The first is the introduction of commercially prepared and sterilized goods of all kinds. The second is the setting up of Central Sterile Supply Departments or C.S.S.D.s as they are usually called, in which dressings, theatre clothing and instruments are serviced, packed and sterilized for use in all parts of the hospital. The third is the provision of somewhat similar central departments in which the highly specialized equipment required for anaesthesia, artificial respiration, dialysis and similar procedures can be prepared and sterilized.

Because of these developments, a nurse may never be called upon at any stage in her training to prepare and sterilize anything required in operating theatres, wards or out-patient departments. Nevertheless, there are still many parts of the world where some if not all of these new facilities are not available because of financial stringency, distance from sources of supply or such extreme isolation that essential public services such as gas or electricity are not available. If therefore sterilization is required, the nurse may have to take charge herself. In addition to this she may also have to play an active part in deciding what methods should be used for the procedures that are required for the prevention of cross or hospital acquired infection. Because of these commitments, she may be compelled to employ methods with which she has had little previous experience.

But in view of the fact that the methods that are required in one situation may be very different from those required in others, it is advisable to give some indication of what can be done in these circumstances.

Air. In general, it is impracticable to attempt to remove organisms from air, but that which is forced into operating theatres by fans generally passes through filters which abstract most of the organisms suspended in it. Such filters require frequent renewal or cleaning because they become choked.

The amount of air forced into the theatre per hour, the design and placing of the inlets, etc., are still matters for debate and are too technical for this book.

Anaesthetic apparatus. The treatment of the relatively elaborate apparatus required nowadays poses special problems that have not been satisfactorily solved and which it would be pointless to debate. Suffice it to say that as much of the apparatus as possible, that is to say, metal parts, corrugated tubing and masks should be autoclaved or pasteurized. Particular attention should be given to humidifiers because *Pseudomonas* can multiply in water and so contaminate the whole apparatus.

Baths. Various methods have been employed for the treatment of baths after use. Perhaps the most important point is the removal of scum. This requires a detergent. It may be combined with an antiseptic containing chlorine.

Bedding. In general, the bedding employed in hospitals does not need special treatment. But it may convey infection to other patients if it has come from a patient with an infectious disease or it has become soiled with urine or faeces. In such a situation, disposable sheets and pillow cases can be employed. If they are not available, the linen or cotton articles should be placed in an impervious bag which can be completely sealed. The contents can then be placed direct without handling, into water at 70°C for at least half an hour by which time, the pathogens should have been killed and they can be laundered in the usual way. Immersion of the articles in an antiseptic solution is much less satisfactory.

Cotton blankets can be treated in the same manner as sheets but those made of wool pose special problems because they become very heavy when wet and are difficult to dry. If therefore, it is essential to treat them, they can be autoclaved or exposed to formalin vapour.

Mattresses and pillow cases are even more difficult to deal with for which reason the most satisfactory method of all is not to attempt their sterilization but to enclose them in plastic covers which can be wiped down with an antiseptic. If this has not been done, the only recourse is autoclaving or exposure to formalin vapour.

Bedpans. Disposable bedpans have many advantages but they are expensive and require a special machine to deal with them. Metal bedpans are best dealt with by an apparatus that empties, washes and treats them with steam in one operation. This too, may not be available in which case they must be emptied, washed with water and if possible, sterilized in an autoclave. Treatment with antiseptics cannot be recommended and should be avoided if possible.

In whatever way they are treated, they should be delivered to the patient in a paper bag into which they should be placed after use.

Catheters. Whenever possible, disposable ready sterilized plastic catheters should be used, but if they are not available, rubber catheters can be sterilized by boiling. So too can those made of gum elastic but the later must be placed at once into cold water in order to harden them.

Crockery and cutlery. Any pathogenic organisms likely to be present will be killed if they are washed thoroughly in water whose temperature is over 60°C. Washing machines ensure this. But if they are not available, care must be taken that the temperature of the water is high enough. Provided they are disposed of after use, plastic cutlery and paper cups and plates can be employed.

Cystoscopes, sigmoidoscopes and bronchoscopes. Because they contain lenses and electrical elements, such instruments must be specially treated. If suitable apparatus is available, they can be sterilized by ethylene oxide gas. Failing this, the most satisfactory method would appear to be 'pasteurization' in which the instrument is placed in water at a temperature of 75°C for 30 minutes. If this is not possible the only alternative is to dismantle the instrument and boil or autoclave those parts that would not be harmed in the process and immerse the remainder in an antiseptic solution.

Dressings, drapes and gowns. It is usually possible to obtain these articles ready sterilized in paper or cloth wrappings from commercial sources or a C.S.S.D. If not, they must be packed and sterilized by steam in an autoclave employing the method described on page 105.

Faeces. The treatment of faeces from normal persons has already been discussed on page 85. That of patients with an intestinal infection requires rather more drastic treatment. The faeces must be rendered free of pathogens by treatment for an hour with a strong antiseptic such as Sudol diluted 1/10. In poliomyelitis, Chloros 1/20 should be employed.

Feeding bottles and *teats*. After use, they should be thoroughly washed. The teats should be rubbed with salt to remove traces of milk. Preferably, both bottles and teats should then be boiled, pasteurized or autoclaved. An alternative is total immersion in a chlorine containing antiseptic such as Milton 1/80 for at least two hours, followed by washing to remove the antiseptic.

Fluids. The glucose, saline and similar fluids required for intravenous injection should be autoclaved in a container constructed in such a way that the contents can be delivered direct into a vein.

Those intended for irrigation should be autoclaved in bottles with a cap that acts as a protective device preventing contamination of the fluid when being poured out.

Gloves. Disposable ready sterilized gloves are by far the best. But if they cannot be obtained and rubber gloves must be used, it is of some importance that they cannot be sterilized in an autoclave at the same temperature as that employed for dressings etc., because they become brittle and virtually unusable. This is due to the harmful effect of the hot dry air which comes into contact with them in the drying process of the autoclave cycle. If however they are sterilized in a modern theatre autoclave using steam at a temperature of 132°C for 5 minutes, the steam removed by vacuum pump, replaced by air and the containers containing the gloves removed at once, they need not be damaged.

When such an installation is not available the only alternative is to autoclave at 115°C or 10 lb pressure for 30 minutes.

Incubators for premature infants. Because of their method of construction many cannot be sterilized in the ordinary sense of the term. All that can be done is to wipe them down with an antiseptic such as Milton or Chloros 1/100.

Instruments, bowls and trays. For many purposes, the disposable, commercially packed and sterilized instruments such as forceps and knives are by far the most convenient. But the larger instruments still cannot be obtained in this way. Before sterilization is attempted, they should be thoroughly cleaned, particular attention being paid to the hinges of scissors and similar situations in which dirt, blood, pus, etc. may have remained after previous use. All particles of grease must also be removed because water or steam cannot penetrate to reach the metal underneath.

Several methods can be employed for the actual sterilization. By far the best is autoclaving with live steam. In operating theatres, small automatically operated autoclaves using steam at as high a temperature as 132°C which require only 3 minutes to effect complete sterilization are frequently employed. With such equipment it is not necessary to wrap the articles; they can be placed direct on the instrument table.

If the instuments will not be used at once, they must be packed in a suitable manner, placed in containers autoclaved as described on page 104.

Autoclaves suitable for hospitals are not usually available in clinics or the consulting rooms of general practitioners but a good domestic pressure cooker set to work at 15 lb per square inch will also serve. Apparatus of this description can be used for the sterilization of small instruments and dressings that are not too bulky.

There remain, however, many situations in medical practice where even the simplest and cheapest equipment of this description is still not available. In this event, the only recourse is the use of boiling water. The apparatus and methods that should be employed for this purpose have already been described on pages 102–103 and need not be repeated.

Knives and suture needles. Although ready sterilized knife blades and needles can generally be obtained everywhere, if such be not the case, they must be autoclaved or boiled in water, particular care being taken to guard the cutting edges by their being held in clips on pieces of metal or wrapped in lint.

Mechanical ventilators. These are even more difficult to deal with than anaesthetic apparatus but the same methods should be employed. Here too, special attention should be paid to the humidifiers; those on some machines can be pasteurized.

Napkins. The ideal is to use disposable napkins which, after removal, can be placed in an impervious bag and burnt. But as they are expensive and may not even be obtainable in many parts of the world, the only alternative is the conventional cotton square which must be washed and used again. Immediately after use, they should be placed in a receptacle, preferably a bin containing antiseptic at the side of the cot. The contents of these bins can be emptied into a common receptacle which is kept in the sluice room. This must also contain antiseptic. The napkins can then be washed, but if possible this should not be done in the ward or nursery or by someone who prepares feeding bottles. These processes should take place somewhere else and preferably by a method which involves their being boiled. Great care must be taken that they do not subsequently come into contact with soiled napkins or be returned to the ward in containers that have been used for them.

Skin. Since the skin of the hands of the surgeon and that of an operation site on the patient may be contaminated by pathogenic organisms, an attempt must be made to remove as many as possible. Washing alone may suffice for this but there is always danger that they may re-appear after a time from the hair follicles and sweat glands. These can only be dealt with by the application of antiseptics following the washing process Iodophers or chlorexidine may be employed.

Sputum. This is best collected in screw capped disposable plastic containers.

Suture materials. Catgut requires special methods for sterilization so that it can only be obtained ready prepared in glass containers. Other materials such as silk, linen or nylon can also be purchased ready sterilized in peel back foil or plastic containers. If they cannot be obtained in this form, silk and linen thread can be wound loosely on spools, boiled or autoclaved and stored in a sterile dry container. Man-made fibres such as Terylene and nylon can be boiled but must not be autoclaved. They too are best preserved dry.

Syringes. Commercially sterilized syringes and needles are employed. Hot air sterilization of glass syringes which was used in the past is now no longer carried out

Thermometers. Each patient should have his own thermometer which is kept entirely separate from the others. When the patient has been discharged, thorough washing will usually suffice but if it appears advisable, it may be treated with an antiseptic such as 70 per cent alcohol containing 1 per cent iodine.

Tubing. Commercially sterilized disposable polythene tubing is used. The tubing used in anaesthesia is often pasteurised (see p. 103). Care must be taken to remove air locks.

Urinals. Disposable urinals are available but they are expensive and take up space. Glass or plastic models should be washed after emptying, and pasteurized usually in a bed pan and urinal washer. The use of antiseptics is not recommended. However some attempt must be made to rid them of their organisms because they can be responsible for cross-infection, particularly in uro-genital wards.

Wards and nurseries. Although potentially pathogenic organisms derived from patients may be present in the air, and on the floor or furniture, it is virtually useless to attempt their eradication for they soon re-appear. For this reason, the treatment of floors and walls with antiseptic solutions, a practice at one time common, is becoming unusual. The most useful measure is to avoid their dissemination into the atmosphere during domestic and other activities by employing a vacuum cleaner for removal of dust and fluff from the floor and a moist rather than a dry duster when dusting.

Much the same applies to single rooms occupied by patients with infectious diseases and when the room is vacated, a thorough cleaning is all that is usually required. But when the room has been occupied by a patient with a highly infectious disease, an attempt should be made to effect terminal disinfection as it is usually called, before the room is occupied by another patient. For this purpose, formalin vapour is usually employed. The windows must first be closed and sealed with adhesive tape, and the chimney, if there is one, blocked. The vapour can be produced by heating tablets or be liberated by pressure from a tank. As soon as the apparatus begins to function the door must be closed and sealed with tape. The vapour should be allowed 24 hours in which to act.

7

Prevention of infection by immunization

It is either impossible or impracticable to prevent many forms of infection by elimination of the sources of the organisms concerned or cutting the lines of communication by which they travel, but prevention is still possible if the human population can be made resistant to infection. This may result from active or passive immunization.

ACTIVE IMMUNIZATION

The term active immunization can be defined as a method of acquiring immunity in which the individual's own cells respond to certain forms of stimulation in such a way that he becomes resistant to infection by a particular micro-organism. It is extremely probable that this resistance is usually due to the formation of antibodies which enable the individual to kill the organism as soon as it reaches him and neutralize the toxins it produces. Such immunity may be acquired as a result of different stimuli.

Clinical infection

It is well known that following recovery from many forms of

infection such as measles, whooping cough, diphtheria, scarlet fever, smallpox, chicken pox, mumps, typhoid fever and poliomyelitis, the patient becomes completely immune, so that, as a rule, he is not likely to suffer a second attack, no matter how long he lives. Nevertheless, this does not follow common colds, influenza and herpes simplex, repeated attacks of all three diseases being the usual experience.

This method of obtaining immunity possesses the obvious disadvantage that it can only be acquired at the cost of an attack of the disease in question. Since many of these diseases can end fatally, and, even when the patient recovers, may produce serious after effects, it is obvious that deliberate exposure to disease in order to obtain immunity cannot be recommended.

Subclinical infection

An almost equally high degree of immunity may also be obtained as a result of subclinical infection. In this, pathogenic organisms settle in the tissues but without necessarily producing all the symptoms of a fully developed clinical infection. But as a result of this, antibodies are produced that can protect the individual against clinical infection. Many people react in this way to such diseases as diphtheria, scarlet fever, poliomyelitis, typhoid, paratyphoid and dysentery. Unfortunately, many pathogens are evidently unable to produce subclinical infection. Those responsible for smallpox, gonorrhoea, syphilis, chickenpox and measles are examples of this.

This method of acquiring immunity also possesses disadvantages. In the first place, it is quite impossible to obtain it purposely for even if one exposed oneself to patients suffering from infection, one cannot predict whether one will suffer nothing more than the almost negligible symptoms of a subclinical attack or be so unfortunate as to go through the miseries of the fully developed infection with its attendant risks of death, or the complications that may ensue even when recovery occurs. In the second place, one can only acquire immunity in this way, if one lives in a commanity in which the organisms in question are producing disease. It is for this reason that it is possible to obtain immunity against typhoid, paratyphoid and diphtheria if one lives in a country such as India in which they are common. But the first two diseases have been virtually eradicated in England as a result of sanitation and the third by immunization, so that very few Englishmen have had subclinical attacks of these diseases and thereby have acquired immunity in this way.

Infection by organisms whose pathogenic abilities have been attenuated

If, as already described in the preceding section, it is possible to obtain lasting immunity as a result of so mild a stimulus as subclinical infection, it is equally possible that this might be brought about artificially; that is to say by producing a very slight infection with organisms whose ability to produce the usual symptoms has been diminished in some way. In general, this is not possible, for most pathogenic organisms administered to human beings would produce the full syndrome of clinical infection. But some have been treated in such a manner that their virulence has diminished to such an extent that they produce few or no symptoms. Such organisms are said to have been *attenuated*. Nevertheless, they can stimulate the immunity apparatus sufficiently to enable the individual to resist infection by the normal virulent strains of the same organism. Suspensions of such attenuated organisms are known as *vaccines* and are used for the prevention of small-pox, tuberculosis, yellow fever, measles and rubella.

Smallpox. Vaccination, as the method of immunization employed to protect against this disease is usually called, was first introduced as long ago as 1795 by Edward Jenner. It

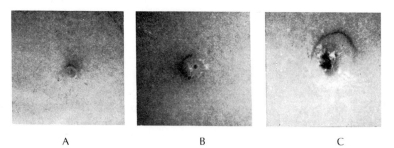

A   B   C

Fig. 7.1 A Primary Take following vaccination. (A) 7th day; (B) 10th day; (C) 12th day.

involves the production of a small, strictly localized area of infection in the skin by a strain of smallpox virus that has become so attenuated by growth for many generations in rabbits or calves, that it is no longer capable of producing smallpox.

As smallpox has been eradicated and vaccination is now only carried out on laboratory workers handling the virus the technique will not be described further.

Tuberculosis. The two Frenchman, Calmette and Guérin, obtained a strain of tubercle bacilli known as B.C.G. (*Bacille Calmette-Guérin*) which is too weak to produce actual tuberculosis but is able to multiply to a very limited extent if injected into the skin of human beings. In doing so, it produces a bluish red papule in about three weeks. The skin over it is thin and shining, while the base may be indurated. It enlarges until it reaches its maximum size in about six weeks. Thereafter it begins to regress. In the more severe reactions, the skin may break down allowing the escape of a serous fluid. Very rarely, an ulcer may form as a result of sloughing of the centre of the papule. But in general, all trace of the lesion has disappeared by the third month and scarring is very unusual.

B.C.G. cannot be given until it has been ascertained whether or not the individual is sensitive to tuberculin. This is a protein which appears in the broth in which tubercle bacilli have grown. Such tests are necessary for two reasons. Individuals who are sensitive to tuberculin would suffer very severe reactions if they were given B.C.G.; and immunization of such persons is not so necessary, for they are much less likely to contract tuberculosis than those who are insensitive to tuberculin.

Tuberculin tests. Tuberculin is a liquid which must be applied to the skin. It can be incorporated in a jelly or in gauze which is then held in contact with the skin for 24 hours. But it is more usual for it to be administered by injection into the deeper layers of the skin as in the Heaf and Mantoux tests.

In the Heaf test, the tuberculin is pricked into the skin at about 8 points by a spring-operated instrument. The strongest solution of tuberculin is alone used and is smeared on the skin beforehand.

The Mantoux test is much less commonly used. 0.1 ml of tuberculin is injected intradermally using a special syringe.

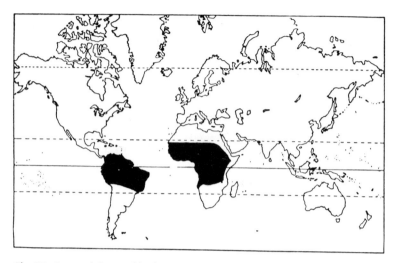

Fig. 7.2 Areas of the world where yellow fever virus and the insect vector responsible for its transmission are still present. Despite this, widespread immunization has almost eradicated the disease.

One unit of tuberculin is used at first and if the reaction with this is negative the dose may be increased to 10 or 100 units. When, as a result of these tests, it is obvious that the individual is insensitive to tuberculin, he can then be given B.C.G. One method is to inject the organisms into the skin, using a syringe of the same pattern as that employed for tuberculin. The dose administered is 0.1 ml and the skin should be cleaned with alcohol, not with an antiseptic.

A second method involves smearing the B.C.G. on the surface of the skin and then driving it into the skin with a spring-actuated apparatus similar to that used for the Heaf test, but which has 20 needle points.

There seems to be little doubt that immunization with B.C.G. is a valuable method of obtaining protection against tuberculosis. It has done much to prevent the disease amongst nurses and others who come into close contact with open cases of acute tuberculosis. It is also being used extensively in countries such as India, where the disease is common and facilities for the isolation and treatment of cases in the infectious stage are almost non-existent. Nevertheless, it should not be given to anyone with localized sepsis or eczema.

Poliomyelitis. This desease can be prevented by the administration of living but attenuated virus known as the Sabin vaccine. It can be incorporated in sweets or in the form of drops on pieces of sugar and in this way reaches the intestinal canal. Here, the virus multiplies but causes no symptoms. As a result, antibodies are formed that persist for several years and protect the patient against the disease. There is no doubt about the value of the procedure. It is however worth remembering that the vaccine should not be given to anyone with a gastrointestinal disturbance or who is known to be sensitive to polymyxin, streptomycin or neomycin, traces of which may be present in the vaccine.

Yellow fever. The virus employed for protection against this disease has become so attenuated that it no longer either produces the disease itself or any local reaction at the site of injection. It is grown in eggs and is issued in the form of a dry powder which must be dissolved before injection. It is given by subcutaneous injection. Immunity to the disease begins to develop after about ten days, and may last for many years thereafter. Since the vaccine is made in eggs, it should not be given to anyone who is sensitive to them or to polymyxin and neomycin.

Measles. Living attenuated measles virus is employed and is of considerable value. It must not be given before the first birthday because maternal antibodies would inactivate it if given sooner. Like some of the other vaccines mentioned above, its employment is contra-indicated for anyone known to be sensitive to eggs, polymyxin or neomycin. But serious consideration may also be required before it is given to children with a history of convulsions, epilepsy and any chronic disease of the heart or lungs.

Rubella. A living attenuated virus vaccine has been developed for protection against the disease. Since the disease itself is so mild, it is not necessary to immunize whole populations but the vaccine should certainly be employed for the prevention of the disease during pregnancy when there is a risk that congenital defects may develop in the foetus. If possible, it should be given before puberty. Whether it should be given after puberty is more controversial, particularly if conception is likely to occur soon afterwards. The reason for this is that the virus in the vaccine is alive and may reach the foetus to produce infection and the congenital defects that can result.

It is, for this reason, only advisable to use the vaccine for older women if pregnancy is avoided for two months afterwards.

Contra-indications peculiar to the use of living vaccines. In addition to the contra-indications mentioned under each of the vaccines discussed above, there are others that apply to all of them. This is largely due to the fact that although they are all apparently harmless, they consist of living organisms which might become dangerous in certain circumstances. For this reason, no two vaccines should be administered at the same time. An interval of three weeks is advisable. Nor should any of them be given to persons whose immunity apparatus is known to be inefficient because of hypogammaglobinaemia, immuno-suppressive therapy or the administration of cortico-steroids. Nor should they be given to anyone with an already active infection particularly when it is sufficiently serious to be accompanied by fever.

Injection of killed organisms

In view of the fact that immunity resulting from clinical infection, subclinical infection, and immunization with attenuated organisms, is probably due to the development of antibodies by the cells of the patient, in response to their stimulation by chemical compounds coming from the organisms growing in the tissues, it is a justifiable assumption that the cells will be stimulated in the same way if the compounds themselves are injected and carried by the blood stream to the cells. The easiest way to obtain these compounds is to grow the organisms and then kill them in such a way that the compounds are not altered. Application of heat or dilute antiseptics can both be employed for this purpose. Like those in which the organisms are still alive, these suspensions are also called *vaccines*.

They are all administered by subcutaneous injection and two are usually required. This is due to the fact that the antibody-producing cells require repeated stimulation to perform their function efficiently so that two doses, given 10–14 days apart, produce much more antibody and therefore better protection than would be the case if both doses are administered at one injection.

They are employed for protection against whooping cough,

typhoid and paratyphoid fevers, cholera, plague, typhus, influenza and rabies.

Typhoid and paratyphoid fevers, cholera, and plague. These consist of suspensions of killed organisms responsible for these diseases. They are not employed as a routine in this or other developed countries where the risk of contracting these diseases is very small. They should be given to anyone about to travel to countries where hygiene is poor and insects such as fleas are common. Two doses are usually required and booster doses every six months for cholera and plague are generally advisable.

Typhus. The organisms responsible for this disease cannot be cultivated on artificial media and it is only by growing them in the cells lining the yolk sac of developing eggs that a suspension can be obtained. Although purified in such a manner that most of the egg proteins are removed, sufficient may remain to cause symptoms if the recipient of the vaccine is allergic to eggs. It should not be given to such persons nor should it be given unless the recipient is going to places where the disease is common, such as Eastern Europe, the Balkans, the Middle East and parts of central America.

Influenza. The vaccine employed consist of a suspension of virus particles grown in the cells of the chrorioallantoic sac of the hen's egg and for this reason may contain sufficient egg protein to produce reactions in anyone allergic to eggs. There is also doubt about its value as a protection against the disease and it is expensive to make. For these reasons it is usual to employ it only for the protection of elderly persons or key personnel who may come into contact with the disease, such as nurses and other workers in hospitals.

Whooping cough. Although this disease is seldom serious or likely to cause death if contracted after the first birthday, it can bring about collapse of the lung, bronchopneumonia and encephalopathy in children who become infected before that time. Because of this, it is one of the most important infective causes of death in young children.

There is no doubt that immunization can protect against this disease provided the first dose is given about the third month of life. But, unfortunately, the vaccine has recently come under suspicion of being the cause of sufficient damage to the central

Table 7.1 Vaccines and toxoids required for prophylactic immunization

Disease	Vaccines employed	No. of doses	Time of administration	Remarks
		I Routine administration to children		
Diphtheria	Toxoid A.P.T.	5	(1) 9 months (2) 10–11 months	Can be given with tetanus and whooping cough vaccines
	P.T.A.P. Floccules		(3) 18–21 months (4) 5 years (5) 8–12 years	
Tetanus	Toxoid	5	(1) 9 months (2) 10–11 months (3) 18–21 months (4) 5 years (5) 8–12 years	Can be given with diphtheria and whooping cough vaccines
Whooping cough	Killed organisms		(1) 9 months (2) 10–11 months (3) 18–21 months	Can be given with diphtheria and tetanus vaccines
Poliomyelitis	Living attenuated virus— Sabin vaccine		(1) 6 months (2) 7 months (3) 15 months (4) 5 years	Vaccine contains penicillin
Measles	Living attenuated virus		16–24 months	Fever and rash fairly common
Tuberculosis	Living B.C.G.	1	10–12 years	Preliminary Mantoux or Heaf test required
Rubella (German measles)	Living attenuated virus		Schoolgirls before puberty Non-immune women of childbearing age	Pregnancy should be avoided for 2 months

II Immunization of intending travellers

Cholera	Killed organisms	2 with interval of 28 days	Before going to endemic areas	Booster every 6 months
Yellow fever	Living attenuated virus	1	Before going to endemic areas	Immunity lasts 5 years
Typhoid and Para-typhoid A, B, and C	Killed organisms	2 with interval of 28 days	Before going to endemic areas	Reactions common
Typhus	Killed organisms	2 with interval of 10 days	Before going to endemic areas	Booster annually
Plague	Killed organisms	2 with interval of 1–3 weeks	Before going to endemic areas	Booster every 6 months

III Immunization of adults

Influenza	Killed virus		Before an epidemic	For susceptible individuals and key workers

nervous system of some children to bring about mental retardation or epilepsy when the child grows up.

It is advisable to withhold the vaccine from children with a history of convulsions, cerebral irritation, or who come from families in which there is a history of epilepsy or other diseases of the central nervous system. Nor should it be given to children with developmental neurological defects and not until the child has recovered if there is any febrile illness particularly of the respiratory tract.

There has recently been a considerable increase in the number of cases of whooping cough in children in the British Isles. This follows a decrease in the uptake of immunization because of anxiety about the side effects of the vaccine. Because these side effects are rare and because whooping cough is a severe disease in young children parents are advised that apart from exceptional circumstances children should be immunized.

Rabies. This too is a suspension of virus particles. Previously the virus was grown in duck eggs but now human embryo lung cells are being used. The employment of this vaccine is also limited. Prophylactically it can be used for the protection of kennel maids and veterinarians who may come into contact with rabid dogs in the course of their duties. But unlike the vaccines so far referred to, this vaccine can be employed to prevent development of the disease in people who have been bitten by a rabid dog. The incubation period of rabies may be so long that if immunization starts as soon after the bite as possible immunity to the disease may develop sufficiently soon to prevent the development of the disease.

Following the administration of some vaccines, particularly those employed for protection against typhoid and paratyphoid, local reactions with swelling and redness of the skin may occur within 24 hours of the injection. Generalized symptoms comprising headache, nausea, vomiting and a rise in temperature may also occur. They are of no importance and soon subside.

Injection of toxoid

In two diseases, diphtheria and tetanus, the organisms remain localized at the point of entry and most of the symptoms are due to the liberation of a powerful exotoxin by the organisms.

But if the individual has sufficient antibody (usually referred to as an antitoxin) in his circulating blood, it will neutralize the toxins as soon as they are formed. As a result, the patient will not suffer from most of the symptoms of the disease in question, even if the organisms are present in the tissues.

The necessary antibody will appear in the circulating blood if a series of injections of toxin have been previously administered. Unfortunately, toxin is too dangerous for this purpose. A modified form of toxin known as *toxoid*, however, acts in exactly the same way but is completely harmless. It is made by adding formalin to the toxin (which is present in the liquid part

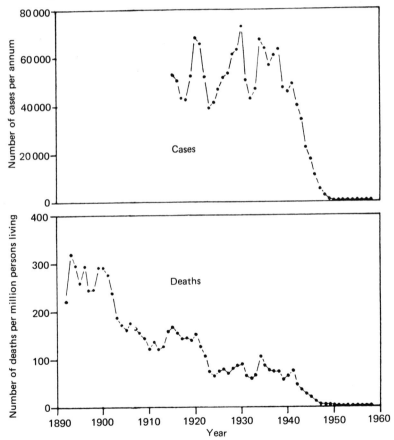

Fig. 7.3 Abrupt fall in the number of cases and deaths per annum from diphtheria in England and Wales following widespread immunization in 1941 and the succeeding years.

of a broth culture of the organisms) and incubating the mixture for about a month. Toxoids made in this way are used for immunization against diphtheria and tetanus.

Diphtheria. Liquid toxoid, made as described above, can be used alone but it is more usual for it to be combined with something else to improve its immunizing properties. Alum can be employed for this purpose and the combination is known as *Alum precipitated toxoid* or A.P.T. A second substance is aluminium phosphate in which case it is referred to as *Purified toxoid on aluminium phosphate* or P.T.A.P. Thirdly, the toxoid may be mixed with antitoxin and the precipitate that appears is employed for immunization. This is known as *Toxoid antitoxin floccules* or T.A.F. Liquid toxoid can also be combined with a suspension of whooping cough bacilli so that injection of the mixture will produce protection against both diphtheria and whooping cough. This reduces the number of injections that must be given in childhood.

Whatever material is employed it is of great importance that at least two doses and with liquid toxoid, three, be given. The intervals between injections should be 4–6 weeks or even longer.

It is desirable that all children should be immunized during the first year of life. But because the immunity produced may not persist, it is necessary that single *booster doses* be given when the child first goes to school, again when it reaches its tenth or eleventh birthday and if possible when it leaves school.

As a general rule, adults are not immunized but if it is necessary to do so, it is important to determine whether or not they already possess antitoxin as a result of previous clinical or subclinical infection because immunization of such individuals is not only unnecessary but severe reactions may occur. The Schick test is employed for this purpose.

Schick test. Diluted toxin in a dose of 0.2 ml is injected intradermally in the front of the forearm. No reaction is produced if the individual already possesses sufficient antitoxin to neutralize the toxin injected. If he has no antitoxin, a red flush 1 to 5 cm in diameter begins to develop within 24–48 hours. It gradually becomes more obvious and is at its height on the third or fourth day.

Because somewhat similar changes may occur if the individual is sensitive to the proteins which are invariably present in the test solution in addition to the toxin, it is necessary to inject a control solution into the skin of the other arm. This may consist of toxin that has been boiled to inactivate it. In America, toxoid is used for this purpose.

In general, Schick testing is unnecessary with children under the age of ten but it is advisable when anyone above that age is being immunized for the first time. One reason is that he may have become immune so that immunization is unnecessary, and the second is that quite severe reactions may occur even when the individual is immune.

Recently determination of serum antitoxin levels has begun to replace Schick testing as a method of assessing immunity to diphtheria.

There is no doubt whatever of the value of immunization against diphtheria. Prior to 1941 there were usually between 40 000 and 50 000 cases of the disease every year in England and Wales. Following widespread immunization in that year and in the succeeding years, the number of cases has steadily fallen. So much so that in 1957 it was only 37 and in 1958, 78. The same low rates still prevail.

Tetanus. The liquid toxoid can be used to prevent the disease but recently, toxoid combined with alum has been introduced. The liquid toxoid can be mixed with other agents such as whooping cough vaccine or diphtheria toxoid. No tests resembling the Schick test are required, largely because there is reason to believe that no one is naturally immune to the disease.

When the liquid toxoid is employed, three doses of 1 ml each at intervals of 4–6 weeks or even longer must be given. Only two doses are necessary when using toxoid combined with alum. Booster doses at intervals of 5 years are also advisable. Whenever possible, children should be immunized in this way, partly because they are more likely to get the disease than adults and partly because it will not be necessary to give them anti-tetanus serum if they hurt themselves. Adults who are particularly prone to the disease, such as men in the armed forces, sportsmen, demolition and agricultural workers, should also be immunized.

There is also evidence that following a booster dose of toxoid, the individual may become hypersensitive to the toxoid for which reason no further booster doses should be given during the next twelve months.

There is no doubt about the value of these procedures. For example, all American troops were immunized against tetanus in the second world war and there was only one case amongst 160 250 battle casualties instead of the 1000 or 2000 that would have probably occurred had there been no immunization of any kind.

PASSIVE IMMUNIZATION

Passive immunization can be defined as a method of obtaining immunity in which the antibodies required have come from another person or animal. It may be acquired naturally or artificially.

Naturally acquired

At the time of birth the child usually has the same antibodies in its blood as those of its mother, probably because the maternal antibodies can traverse the placenta. As most women of childbearing age have already had such diseases as measles, mumps and chickenpox during childhood, it follows that the antibodies she produced to cure herself and which she still possesses render the newborn child as immune to these diseases as she is. Unfortunately, this immunity does not last very long because the antibodies acquired from the mother have usually disappeared by the time of the child's first birthday; but as long as they persist they are of undoubted value to the child.

Artificially acquired

Antibodies can be obtained from human beings or suitably immunized animals. Those coming from human beings are administered in the form of *gamma* globulin. This invariably contains antibodies for measles virus and can accordingly be used to protect young children against this disease. It also contains antibodies for hepatitis virus and can be used for the protection of individuals going to places such as India where the disease is common.

Antibodies derived from animals have generally been produced as a result of a long series of injections of toxin or toxoid into large animals such as horses or oxen. When the antibodies have made their appearance blood is taken and allowed to clot. The serum is then processed so that unwanted constituents such as the albumen are removed and the antibodies themselves are concentrated into a small volume of fluid.

As a general rule, the antibodies produced in this way are employed for the neutralization of toxins and are therefore referred to as *antitoxins*. They have two important disadvantages. They do not persist for very long after their injection and have virtually disappeared in ten to fourteen days. It may therefore be necessary to repeat the injection. Secondly, they are, so far as human beings are concerned, a foreign protein and may cause anaphylaxis if administered to sensitive individuals, particularly those who have received previous injections of antitoxin. But in spite of these drawbacks, antitoxins are undoubtedly of value in certain circumstances.

Tetanus antitoxin. In the past, 500 to 1500 units of tetanus antitoxin or A.T.S. in three doses at weekly intervals was administered to almost all patients with traumatic wounds. But because a high proportion of the population is already protected by previous immunization with toxoid, and severe and even fatal anaphylactic shock may follow its administration, the use of A.T.S. is now restricted to those who have never received toxoid and who have severe and dirty wounds. If anti-tetanus serum is given, human serum is now generally used. There are far fewer reaction to this than to the horse serum previously used.

Tetanus antitoxin is of very doubtful value for the treatment of the disease itself.

Diphtheria antitoxin. As with tetanus, it is possible to prevent diphtheria by injection of antitoxin. It is usually employed to protect children who have been exposed to the disease. The dose usually recommended for this purpose is 500 to 20 000 units given subcutaneously.

Unlike tetanus, diphtheria can be successfully treated by antitoxin. For mild cases a dose of 8000–10 000 units may suffice, but for more serious cases, particularly if they are not seen until the third day or after, 30 000 or even 100 000 units should be given. If possible the antitoxin should be given intravenously. There is no doubt whatever of its value but it is of great importance that it be administered as soon as possible after the development of the disease. The death rate in cases treated on the first day may be only 2–4 per cent, whereas it may be as high as 25–28 per cent amongst cases where treatment is delayed to the seventh day.

Antitoxins in gas gangrene. Antitoxin capable of neutralizing the toxins of gas gangrene bacilli can be employed for the prevention of the disease following severe traumatic wounds or operations on areas of the body where the blood supply is poor. But prophylactic penicillin is probably of more value.

Antitoxin in botulism. An antitoxin which neutralizes the toxin produced by the bacillus responsible is now available and is recommended for the treatment of the disease. It must be added that the disease may be difficult to diagnose and treatment may, therefore, be initiated much too late.

Antirabies serum. Serum containing antibodies preventing growth of the virus is now available. It should be given as soon as possible following the bite of the animal suspected of having the disease.

Administration of vaccines, toxoids and antitoxins

The materials to be injected should have been stored in such a way that their potency has not diminished. This usually involves their being kept in a refrigerator. Nor should they be used after the date of expiry. It is also advisable to ascertain the correct dosage from the label or the enclosed literature, because improvements are constantly being introduced that may necessitate unannounced alterations in dosage.

Subcutaneous injections are usually given in the outer aspect of the upper arm. But antisera are sometimes injected subcutaneously into the abdomen.

It is not proposed to describe the technique employed for the injections because it can only be learned by demonstration and practice. But since immunization—particularly of children—frequently occurs in clinics when large numbers must receive injections, certain precautions must be observed.

Because of the possibility that a syringe and needle may become contaminated by hepatitis virus from the blood of a person to whom an injection has been given, a fresh sterile syringe and needle must be provided for each person. By far the most convenient are the disposable articles now available.

In addition to syringes it is also necessary to provide antiseptics and sterile swabs to clean the rubber caps of vials or the necks of ampoules before use. It is debatable whether it is essential to treat the skin before the injection but if considered necessary, alcohol is usually employed.

Active immunization. In general, vaccines and toxoids are employed for the routine immunization of children or for travellers going to countries where certain diseases are either endemic or may appear at any time. Those used for this purpose are given in Table 7.1.

Many countries require the production at the time of entry of valid certificates stating that the traveller has been immunized against certain diseases, particularly cholera and yellow fever. Yellow fever vaccine can only be administered in special centres usually in the larger cities and if possible the necessary injections should be given some time before departure.

In regard to immunization against other diseases, too much depends on the countries likely to be visited and the amount of contact the intending traveller will have with their microorganisms to allow adequate discussion in this book. But suffice it to say that diseases such as tuberculosis, poliomyelitis, typhoid and paratyphoid fevers are still sufficiently common in many subtropical and tropical countries to warrant intending visitors taking the trouble to have themselves immunized if time permits.

Passive immunization. Except possibly for the treatment of diphtheria and the prevention of rabies, tetanus and hepatitis passive immunization by the injection of antibody containing sera is unusual at the present time. But if it is necessary, it must not be forgotten that antisera prepared in animals may produce an anaphylactic reaction (see page 41). This is more likely to occur if the patient has a history of asthma or hay fever or has been given antiserum in the past. For this reason, it is advisable to ascertain whether such a patient is likely to react by injecting a small dose subcutaneously and waiting thirty minutes to see whether symptoms of anaphylaxis make their appearance. If they do not, the full dose may be injected. The use of antisera prepared in animals has decreased considerably in recent years.

8

Treatment of infection

When infection by micro-organisms develops, a whole series of measures must be taken to ensure that the patient has the best possible chance of recovery. Most of them play little part in combating the organisms themselves and for this reason do not concern this book, but some, involving the use of chemical compounds which can kill or prevent the growth of the micro-organisms, are obviously of bacteriological importance.

Such compounds can be employed in two ways—by *local application* to the more accessible parts of the body; and by *parenteral administration* in which they reach the infected area by way of the blood stream following their injection in another part of the body or their absorption from the alimentary canal.

Local application. This method of treatment can be employed when the organisms are present on exposed areas of the body such as the eyes, the mucous membranes of the nose, throat or mouth, the skin and the tissues laid bare by wounds.

Antiseptics are widely used for this purpose. The stronger antiseptics such as phenol and Lysol or those consisting of mercury compounds in the form of perchloride or biniodide have long been recognized to be much too poisonous for this purpose. But milder antiseptics that have a more selective action, being more likely to kill organisms that harm the tissues, have been used a great deal. These include the yellow dyes of the flavine series, chlorine-containing solutions such as eusol and Dakin's fluid or powders containing iodoform and hexachlorophane. Many other proprietary antiseptics, suitably diluted, are also employed in the hope of killing organisms on the nasopharyngeal mucous membrane or in open wounds. There is, however, considerable doubt whether, in fact, the local application of antiseptics is of sufficient value to warrant their employment. When applied to mucous membranes, they are not only diluted by the local secretions, but may be quenched by the protein contained in them. Serum and exudate from open wounds may similarly dilute or inactivate them, but perhaps their most serious defect is their inability to penetrate into the deeper layers of the mucous membranes or the depths of open wounds to deal with the organisms sheltering in these situations. If therefore, good results follow the use of antiseptics, they are probably not due to destruction of the organisms but to the cleansing action of the fluid in which the antiseptic is dissolved. As a result, pus and dried exudate are removed and the flow of lymph to the infected area is promoted.

Antibiotics can also be employed for local application and because they are relatively harmless, high concentrations can be used. They are particularly valuable for infections of the eyes.

Parenteral administration. This may be defined as a method of treatment in which the compound is brought to the organisms by the blood stream from the alimentary canal or an injection site elsewhere in the body. Antiseptics are much too poisonous for use in this way but many other compounds are available which are virtually harmless to the patient in spite of the fact that they may have marked effects on microorganisms. They are usually referred to as *chemotherapeutic agents.*

CHEMOTHERAPEUTIC AGENTS

The most important of the chemotherapeutic agents now available are the *antibiotics.* They are nearly all produced by certain species of moulds or bacteria while growing in a liquid medium. The micro-organisms are removed by filtration and the fluid is treated in such a way that everything but the anti-biotic is removed. As a result, a highly concentrated solution of antibiotic is obtained.

Penicillin was the first antibiotic to be discovered. It was found by Sir Alexander Fleming in cultures of the fungus called *Penicillium notatum*. A suitable method for concentrating and purifying it was worked out by Sir Ernst Chain and Sir Howard Florey demonstrated its value for the treatment of infections.

The second antibiotic to be discovered was streptomycin. Dr Selman Waksman showed that it was present in cultures of a soil organism called *Streptomyces griseus*. Since then, many other antibiotics have been discovered. They include chlor-amphenicol, neomycin, the tetracyclines and nystatin.

Many sulphur-containing compounds known collectively as *sulphonamides* act in very much the same way as the anti-biotics. The first found to be of value was discovered by Dr G. Domagk and named Prontosil. Then came sulphanilamide and sulphapyridine. None of these compounds is now used, partly because they produce undesirable reactions and partly because others, closely resembling them, have been found to be much more powerful. These include sulphathiazole and sul-phadiazine, which are of considerable value in infections by cocci, sulphaguanidine used for infections of the intestinal tract, and the sulphones, employed for leprosy. The more important compounds of this nature that can be used for treat-ment are listed in Table 8.1

None of these compounds can act on all the micro-organisms that are pathogenic for human beings. Some, such as the tetracyclines, have a wide spectrum of activity as it is called, being able to act on organisms so dissimilar as staphylococci the bacilli of undulant fever and some of the rickettsiae, whereas other compounds, of which isoniazide hydrochloride is an example, are only of value in infections by the tubercle bacillus. In spite of their limitations, the introduction of these chemotherapeutic agents within the past twenty years has completely revolutionized the treatment of infections.

Table 8.1 Compounds employed for the chemotherapy of diseases due to micro-organisms

Compound	Chief indications	Side effects
Penicillins Considerable number, some produced by substitution on penicillin nucleus		
Penicillin G	Streptococcal and pneumococcal infections. Gonorrhoea. Gas gangrene. Endocarditis	Hypersensitivity may be produced
Penicillin V	Mild streptococcal infection	Hypersensitivity may be produced
Ampicillin	Bronchitis and other infections due to Gram-negative bacilli such as *Proteus*, *Haemophilus*, coliform, typhoid and paratyphoid bacilli	Hypersensitivity may be produced
Carbenicillin	*Pseudomonas* infections.	Hypersensitivity may be produced
Cloxacillin	Antibiotic resistant staphylococcal infections	Hypersensitivity may be produced
Cephalosporins Resemble penicillins	Urinary tract infections, and a wide variety of other infections	Occasional rashes
Anti-staphylococcal antibiotics Clindamycin	Staphylococcal infections when there is a poor blood supply such as bone. *Bacteroides* infection	Diarrhoea
Fucidin	Staphylococcal infections	Few
Erythromycin	Staphylococcal and streptococcal infections	Few
Vancomycin	Severe staphylococcal infections not responding to other therapy	Severe side effects regularly occur

Table 8.1 (continued)

Compound	Chief indications	Side effects
Broad spectrum antibiotics Act on a wide range of organisms including rickettsiae and chlamydiae		
Tetracyclines	Many diseases including bronchitis, brucellosis, urinary infections and those due to rickettsiae, spirochaetes and chlamydiae	Disorders of the alimentary tract. Staining of teeth if given in early childhood. Liver damage in pregnancy
Chloramphenicol	Acute typhoid fever. *Haemophilus* meningitis	Aplasia of bone marrow
Aminoglycosides Streptomycin. See drugs for tuberculosis		
Neomycin	Only used topically on skin and in the bowel	Toxic for ear and kidney
Gentamicin	Staphylococcal and a wide variety of infections due to Gram-negative bacilli	Toxic for ear and kidney
Peptide antibiotics Bacitracin	Only used for skin infections	Too toxic for parenteral use
Polymyxin	*Pseudomonas* infections Now little used	Toxic for kidney
Synthetic compounds Sulphonamides	Used in combination with trimethoprim	Rashes Renal and bone marrow damage
Trimethoprim	Infections of respiratory and urinary tracts	Few side effects occasional nausea and

Nitrofurantoin	Urinary tract infection	Occasional gastro-intestinal upsets
Nalidixic acid	Urinary tract infection	Occasional nausea and rashes
Metronidazole	Infections due to anaerobic organisms	Nausea, rashes, CNS symptoms
Drugs for treatment of tuberculosis		
Rifampicin	All forms of tuberculosis	A variety of side effects
Isoniazid	All forms of tuberculosis	Insomnia, peripheral neuritis, psychosis
Ethambutol	All forms of tuberculosis	Retrobulbar neuritis. Patients should be warned of this risk
Other drugs include pyrazinamide, streptomycin and para aminosalicylic acid		
Drugs for treatment of leprosy		
Sulphones	Leprosy but prolonged treatment necessary	
Drugs for treatment of fungal infections		
Nystatin	Locally for infection by *Candida*	
Griseofulvin	Athlete's foot and ringworm	Occasional rashes and headaches
Amphotericin	Generalized severe infections	Commonly toxic producing fever, nausea, phlebitis and anaemia
5-Fluorocytosine	Systemic candidiasis	Leucopenia Liver damage
Miconazole	Systemic candidiasis	Few side effects

MAJOR GROUPS OF ANTIBIOTICS

Penicillins

The penicillins are a very useful group of antibiotics, with few side effects apart from hypersensitivity reactions. A great variety of penicillins are available; these are made by the substitution of different side chains on the penicillin nucleus. Some penicillins such as benzyl penicillin (penicillin G) are split by the action of β lactamase, a penicillinase produced by some bacteria although other penicillins are more resistant to its action. The important penicillins include benzyl penicillin (penicillin G), phenoxymethyl penicillin (penicillin V), ampicillin, carbenicillin and cloxacillin. Their main uses are given in Table 8.1. Recently a new compound, clavulanic acid has been introduced. This inhibits penicillinase and it can therefore be used in combination with a penicillinase sensitive penicillin, for the treatment of infections due to penicillinase producing organisms.

Cephalosporins

The cephalosporin nucleus is rather similar to that of penicillin and in the same way as with the penicillins a range of different products have been produced by the substitution of different side chains. There are few toxic effects but some compounds are nephrotoxic and some hypersensitivity reactions may occur.

A large number of new cephalosporins have recently been produced and the choice of the best cephalosporin in a particular situation may be difficult. The early cephalosporins were all given by intramuscular injection; these included cephalothin and cefazolin. Later oral cephalosporins such as cephalexin and cephradine were introduced and also beta-lactamase resistant cephalosporins of which cefamandole, cefoxitin and cefotaxine are examples.

Anti-staphylococcal antibiotics

Erythromycin

Erythromycin is a very safe antibiotic used mainly for the treatment of streptococcal infections. More recently its use has been extended to the treatment of Legionnaire's disease and of campylobacter infections.

Clindamycin

This antibiotic is in addition to its action against Gram-positive cocci is also effective against anaerobes. Its use has declined due to a serious side effect, pseudomembranous colitis. This does occur with other antibiotics but is probably more common with clindamycin.

Fusidic acid

The use of fusidic acid is mainly in the treatment of staphylococcal infections of bones into which it penetrates well.

Vancomycin

The indication for the use of vancomycin is a severe staphylococcal infection resistant to other forms of treatment and its use for this purpose has recently increased. This is in spite of its being regularly toxic and causing thrombophlebitis, pyrexia and damage to the ear.

Broad spectrum antibiotics

Although some of the penicillins and cephalosporins are active against a wide range of organisms in this group we include tetracycline and chloramphenicol which as well as being effective against Gram-positive and Gram-negative organisms also have activity against chlamydiae and rickettsiae.

Chloramphenicol

Because it occasionally causes aplasia of the bone marrow chloramphenicol is used infrequently. It is still valuable, however, for the treatment of haemophilus meningitis, acute typhoid fever and occasionally for severe infections which would otherwise be difficult to treat.

Tetracyclines

These are used for respiratory tract infections particularly chronic bronchitis and in the treatment of acne. The side effects include staining of the deciduous teeth and for this reason they should not be given to children under 7 years of age. There may be overgrowth of resistant organisms in the gut, particularly of candida and if renal function is already impaired it may deteriorate further.

Aminoglycosides

Gentamicin

The most widely used of the aminoglycosides gentamicin is active against Gram-negative bacilli and staphylococci. It is usually given by intramuscular injection and the dosage must be carefully controlled to achieve levels which are therapeutic but not toxic. Toxicity when it occurs is to the ear and the kidney.

A number of new compounds similar to gentamicin have been introduced. These include amikacin and tobramycin which may be active against gentamicin resistant organisms.

Peptides

These include the polymyxins and bacitracin both now little used because of their toxicity.

Synthetic compounds

Sulphonamides

Sulphonamides are now seldom used except in combination with trimethoprim.

Trimethoprim

This until 1979 was available for use only in combination with sulphamethoxazole but can now be used as a single agent. The problem as to whether trimethoprim is best used in combination with a sulphonamide or alone is not resolved.

Its use is mainly in the treatment of infections of the respiratory and urinary tract.

Nitrofurantoin and nalidixic acid

Both of these compounds are almost entirely used for the treatment of urinary tract infections.

Metronidazole

Metronidazole was used for many years for the treatment of trichomonas infections. Its use has been extended to anaerobic infections and it is now used extensively in the prophylaxis of infection following bowel surgery.

Antituberculous chemotherapy

This is a complex area of chemotherapy which is carried out by physicians with special expertise in the subject. The antibiotics which may be used include: rifampicin, isonicotinic acid hydrazide (INAH), ethambutol, pyrazinamide, streptomycin and para-amino-salicylic acid (P.A.S)

Antifungal antibiotics

Nystatin

This is the most commonly used anti-fungal agent and is effective in the local treatment of candida infections.

Griseofulvin

Griseofulvin is also commonly used and is active against dermatophyte infections.

Systemic antifungals

5-fluorocytosine and miconazole are used inthe treatment of systemic candidiasis. Amphotericin is effective against a wide range of systemic fungal infections but its use is limited by toxicity.

Antiviral agents

The use of antiviral agents is limited. This is due to the difficulty of selectively destroying viruses which multiply within the host cells.

Interferon is potentially useful but experience with it is limited. Amantidine may be of value in influenza. Idoxuridine has been used in herpetic infections and more recently acyclovir has shown considerable promise in the same diseases.

Action of chemotherapeutic agents

The chemotherapeutic agents used in medicine act on micro-organisms in a very different way from the antiseptics. The latter combine with the protoplasm of the organisms and directly kill them, whereas the chemotherapeutic agents interfere with their metabolic activities in such a way that they are unable to grow or to multiply. Inhibited in this way they soon die or are easily dealt with by the normal antibacterial mechanisms of the patient.

Resistance to chemotherapeutic substances

This can be a natural characteristic of organisms or it can be acquired. Natural resistance is a permanent attribute of a great many species of micro-organisms. None of the viruses for example are affected by any of the usual agents employed for the treatment of infections. Some of the bacteria are also unaffected. *Pseudomonas* for example is naturally so resistant to most of the antibiotics that with the exception of polymyxin, gentamicin and carbenicillin they cannot be usefully employed for treatment. So far, no way has been found by which to lessen this resistance.

Acquired resistance by species of organisms that were susceptible before and soon after the introduction of many of the agents now available is common. It takes two forms. One is the production of an enzyme that can destroy the agent before it has an opportunity to act on the organisms. This is the reason why some strains of staphylococci resist penicillin; they produce penicillinase which inactivates it. The second is ability to obtain their foodstuffs for growth and reproduction by a different metabolic pathway from that utilized by susceptible strains of the same organism. It is this alteration in their usual behaviour that is responsible for the emergence of strains of *Strep. pyogenes* that are resistant to the sulphonamides.

Whatever form resistance takes it is usually due to growth of a previously susceptible strain of organism in such low concentrations of the agent that some of the bacterial cells are able to survive and multiply to breed a race of organisms that are not only able to resist the action of full therapeutic concentrations of the agent but retain this property more or less indefinitely thereafter. Ability to become resistant in this way depends to a very large extent on the species of organism and the agent to which it is exposed. Haemolytic streptococci, for example, seldom become resistant to penicillin whereas staphylococci can certainly do so. It is, however, a matter of some importance that in the act of becoming resistant to one chemotherapeutic agent their sensitivity to other agents remains unaltered. But if a strain already resistant to one agent is exposed to the action of another, it may become resistant to the second as well. As a result of this process some strains of staphylococci have become resistant to all the antibiotics that are commonly employed.

Of equal importance is the discovery that a strain of an organism that has become resistant to a particular agent can carry a so-called *transfer factor* which conveys ability to resist to other organisms even when they belong to a different species. This is particularly apt to occur with organisms inhabiting the intestinal tract such as coliform, typhoid, dysentery and food infection bacilli. Important in itself, such a possibility becomes even more so as a result of a complementary discovery that organisms that have become resistant in an animal as a result of treatment with an antibiotic, may find their way to a human being and communicate their resistance to organisms that are potentially pathogenic for human beings.

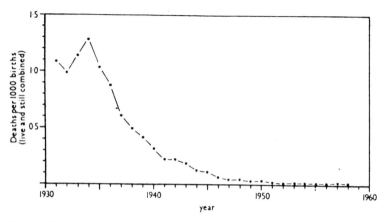

Fig. 8.1 Chemotherapy and its effects. Fall in the death rate from puerperal fever following the introduction of sulphonamides in 1936 and of penicillin in 1946.

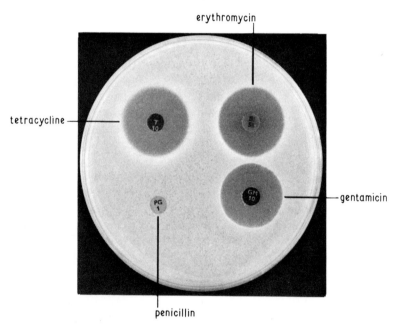

Fig. 8.2 Estimation of the sensitivity of an organism to different antibiotics by filter paper discs. There is growth of the organism everywhere except in zones surrounding the discs containing antibiotics to which the organism is sensitive.

The development of resistance by organisms inhabiting both animals and human beings is of great importance if we are to preserve antibiotics for use in the future. Not only must it be avoided as far as possible, but measures must be taken to prevent dissemination of resistant strains in both human and animal populations. Several measures can be employed to prevent this.

CONTROL OF CHEMOTHERAPY

Adequate dosage. Since resistance may develop when the organisms are exposed to low concentrations of an antibiotic, it follows that full doses must invariably be employed and for a long enough period to ensure that all the infecting organisms have been killed.

Because of the variations on the part of different organisms in their tendency to become resistant, it is impossible to summarize the procedures that should be employed. But, in general, it can be said that while patients usually receive the correct daily dosage, there is a marked tendency for them to discontinue treatment sooner than ordered, particularly when the infection is mild and disappears rapidly.

Use of two chemotherapeutic agents. There are reasons for believing that if full doses of two different agents are given at the same time, the possibility that resistant survivors may be left is very much less than if only one agent is given. In most forms of infection it is unnecessary to use two antibiotics but it is obligatory in the particular case of infection by the tubercle bacillus because of its marked tendency to become resistant to streptomycin the antibiotic usually employed. This should never be given alone.

Prevention of cross infection. Development of resistance on the part of an organism that is causing infection is a serious complication, but the position becomes very much worse if the resistant organism can reach other patients by cross infection. It is largely for this reason that so much attention is being devoted nowadays to the problem of cross infection in hospitals and the methods of preventing it. These have already been discussed in Chapters 3 and 5.

9

The microbiological investigation of disease

A great many diseases may be caused by micro-organisms whose signs and symptoms may range from the severe fulminating infection typified by acute peritonitis to the comparatively minor discomfort associated with a pimple or a boil. Although there is now never any doubt that both diseases are caused by micro-organisms, it was unnecessary for many years to identify the causative organisms, largely because no treatment other than surgical intervention for drainage and the relief of symptoms could be employed. But now that so many infections can be successfully treated by antibiotics and the other chemotherapeutic substances available today, it is frequently imperative to obtain a considerable amount of information if such treatment is likely to be successful. This generally requires answers to three questions.

The first is whether or not the signs and symptoms are, in fact, caused by micro-organisms at all. In many diseases for which they are not responsible, the clinical picture may closely resemble that which is associated with infection. Fever, for example, may be due to heat stroke. Pain and swelling, particularly of a joint, may be due to some form of arthritis which has little or nothing to do with infection. Nausea and vomiting too, although the cardinal signs of food infection can be caused by other agencies than the growth of micro-organisms in the alimentary canal. For reasons such as these it is sometimes essential to employ bacteriological methods in order to ascertain whether the signs and symptoms are, in fact, due to some form of infection.

If then there is no doubt that the illness is an infection, the second question requires an answer. What variety of organism is responsible. This question, too, can sometimes be answered without recourse to bacteriological investigation because the clinical signs in many forms of infection are so distinctive that the organism responsible may not need identification at all. Such is the case when the patient has a boil or stye because both are invariably caused by staphylococci. Certain forms of virus infection of which measles, and chicken pox are examples, do not need usually bacteriological diagnosis for the same reason. Many other diseases are, however, in a very different category. In meningitis for example, almost identical signs and symptoms can be caused by different organisms. Although these organisms are susceptible to treatment by chemotherapy, the drug required for one organism may be quite different from the required for another. Infections in other parts of the body such as the urinary tract and lungs may similarly be caused by different varieties of organisms with corresponding differences in the type of treatment required.

A third question that must be answered is whether or not the microbe is sensitive to the chemotherapeutic substance intended for its treatment. Infections caused by the viruses for example are not usually susceptible to treatment at the present time. But even when the infections are known to be caused by an organism which is usually sensitive, a strain that has become resistant may be responsible. It is, accordingly, frequently necessary to isolate the organism and determine its sensitivity to antibiotics.

Thus, although some forms of infection can be treated quite successfully without the assistance of bacteriological investigations, they may be essential in many others.

Nevertheless, bacteriology has other functions in medical practice than assisting the physician in the diagnosis and treatment of disease. Bacteriological investigations are, for example, frequently required to ascertain the probable source of infection so that further infections can be prevented. They are also employed in hospitals to control the efficiency of the sterilizing procedures employed and in public health laboratories to make certain that water, food and milk are not contaminated by pathogenic organisms.

It is therefore obvious that bacteriology plays an important part in the practice of medicine today. None of the necessary investigations required are the responsibility of the nurse because they require all the resources of a bacteriological laboratory and long experience with its techniques. But the nurse still has a part to play. She may be responsible for the collection of the necessary specimens. She may have to take certain precautions to prevent others becoming infected. She may have to explain matters to anxious relatives and be on the lookout for the complications that may arise. If she is in practice outside a hospital she may have to answer questions about the immunization of children and even act as a mentor on hygiene in the home.

For these reasons, it is advisable for her to have some idea of the diseases themselves, the organisms that cause them, the methods that must be used to isolate and identify them and how the diseases may be prevented and properly treated. The remainder of this chapter and the five chapters that follow deal with these matters.

IDENTIFICATION OF MICRO-ORGANISMS

Both direct and indirect methods are employed for this purpose. *Direct methods.* Microscopic examination of films made from pus, sputum, cerebrospinal fluid, urine, faeces, etc., will frequently enable the bacteriologist to identify the organism responsible. This method is of particular value in meningitis, tuberculosis of the lungs and urinary tract, venereal infections, gas gangrene and ringworm and may be of assistance in pneumonia, diphtheria and in purulent infections.

In these procedures, Gram's stain is of considerable value (see p. 19) and although it is not necessary for a nurse to memorize the reactions of organisms to this method of staining, Table 9.1 shows how organisms behave when stained in this way.

Cultivation of the organisms from the infected area may also assist in making the diagnosis, because it is much easier to

Table 9.1 Differentiation of micro-organisms by Gram's stain

	Gram positive	Gram negative
Cocci	Staphylococci	Gonococci
	Streptococci	Meningococci
	Pneumococci	
Bacilli	Diphtheria bacilli	Coliform bacilli
	Tubercle bacilli	Typhoid bacilli
	Leprosy bacilli	Paratyphoid bacilli
	Gas gangrene bacilli	Food infection bacilli
	Tetanus bacilli	Dysentery bacilli
	Botulism bacilli	*Proteus*
	Anthrax bacilli	*Pseudomonas*
		Haemophilus
		Whooping cough bacilli
		Brucellosis bacilli
		Plague bacilli
		Klebsiella
Vibrio		Cholera vibrio

Spirochaetes, fungi and viruses are not differentiated by Gram's stain.

ascertain the variety responsible, if a culture is available. Nevertheless, the chances of obtaining cultures vary considerably. In purulent infections, diphtheria, meningitis, certain forms of pneumonia, typhoid and paratyphoid, for example, it is quick and relatively easy, whereas in virus infections, it may be very difficult indeed.

As a general rule, cultivation is carried out by spreading some of the infected material over the surface of solid medium in a petri dish and incubating it for 24–28 hours at 37°C. The colonies that develop are frequently so distinctive that it is possible to identify the organism without further investigation. But in some forms of infection, it is necessary to use liquid medium. This is particularly the case when the organism must be cultivated from the circulating blood.

A second and equally important reason for attempting to cultivate the organisms is that this is necessary if properly controlled chemotherapy is contemplated. For this, the sensitivity of the organisms must be determined. Such tests can be carried out in several different ways. One of the easiest is to inoculate the surface of a culture plate with a sufficient number of the organisms to obtain a confluent growth after incubation. Filter paper discs impregnated with known quantities of each of the drugs likely to be employed, are then placed on the surface of the plate.

After the plate has been incubated for 24 hours, the whole of the surface of the medium will be covered by a thin sheet of growing organisms except for zones surrounding the discs containing drugs to which the organisms are sensitive. No such clear zones will be round discs containing drugs to which the organism is insensitive.

Indirect methods. In many infections it may be difficult if not impossible to see the organisms when using the ordinary microscope or to cultivate them in the laboratory on the usual bacteriological media. Nevertheless, it may still be possible to make a diagnosis by indirect methods.

One such method is to ascertain whether antibodies for the organisms suspected of being the cause of the illness have appeared in the circulating blood. This is the basis of the tests used for the diagnosis of syphilis, brucellosis and some other diseases to which further reference is made in the succeeding chapters.

A second method is to ascertain whether the patient has become sensitive or allergic, as it is sometimes called, to the proteins of the organisms suspected of being responsible for the disease. Tests of this nature have sometimes proved useful in the diagnosis of brucellosis, and lymphogranuloma. The method suffers from the disadvantage that this form of sensitivity does not appear until the patient has been ill for some time so that it can only be used in chronic infections.

Most of the diagnostic procedures described above are carried out by experienced laboratory workers. It is important, however, that nurses have some understanding of them so that they can make the best use of the help the laboratory can give. In addition nurses are responsible for obtaining the majority

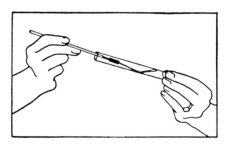

Fig. 9.1 Inoculation of liquid medium.

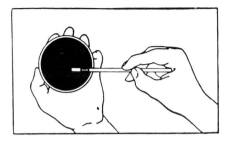

Fig. 9.2 Inoculation of solid medium.

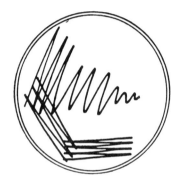

Fig. 9.3 Method of spreading the specimen on the surface of solid medium.

of the specimens sent to the laboratory. They must therefore know how to take the specimens, what materials to use and what precautions to take.

Materials and apparatus required

General. Whatever bacteriological examinations are required, it is essential that the instruments, tubes, swabs and specimen bottles, etc., which come into contact with the specimens, should be sterile and that they should not contain traces of antiseptic.

Swabs. A swab consists of cotton wool wound round the end of a wire or wooden stick and sterilized usually in a plastic tube.

Sterile bottles. Small 25 ml bottles with screw-caps can be used for pus, cerebrospinal fluid, urine or bits of tissue.

Screw capped containers. Made of glass or waxed papier

maché, they can be employed for the collection of sputum, faeces or urine.

Media. As a general rule, the media most suitable for the growth of the organisms likely to be present in the specimen, are inoculated in the laboratory. But in some investigations the media must be inoculated at the bedside or in the clinic. This particularly applies to gonorrhoea, whose causative organism is so sensitive to the action of oxygen and a fall in temperature that it is not likely to survive for very long on an ordinary woollen swab. For this reason, immersion of the swab in a special holding medium in a small bottle is also employed. This keeps the organisms alive until they reach the laboratory.

Labelling. The surname and first name of the patient, his hospital number and the ward, the name of the doctor and the date, together with the provisional diagnosis and investigation required, must be written legibly on the request form. The specimen itself must also be labelled so that it can be matched to the correct request form.

Preservation of specimens in transit

In hospitals the specimen usually finds its way to the laboratory within a reasonable time of its collection from the patient. But it should be realized that, on the whole, bacteria survive better at low than at high temperatures and are very susceptible to direct sunlight. If, therefore, delay in delivery of the specimen is inevitable, it should be placed in a suitable refrigerator. In cases of gonorrhoea or meningitis, it should be kept at room temperature because the organisms responsible are unusual in being sensitive to cold.

OBTAINING SPECIMENS

Mouth. Material for microscopic examination in cases of Vincent's angina or other infections of the mouth can be obtained by rubbing a straight swab over the surface of any ulcers or other infected areas; the tongue must, of course, be kept out of the way.

Throat Specimens should be taken from the surface of the tonsils and the posterior pharyngeal wall, particular care being taken to avoid contamination by mouth organisms. Adequate illumination and a tongue depressor are essential to obtain a good view of the lesions, but the proper technique for taking the specimen can only be learned by experience.

Anterior nares. A straight wooden swab introduced into each of the anterior nares will suffice.

Posterior nares. Two methods can be employed. A thin swab mounted on a flexible wire can be passed through the anterior nares past the turbinate bones into the post-nasal space. A second method is to use a stiff metal swab bent at an angle. This is introduced through the mouth, past the uvula into the post-nasal space.

Sputum. Care must be taken that purulent masses and not saliva are collected for examination. When tuberculosis is suspected, the first expectoration in the morning is the most likely to contain the organism.

Stomach washings. Some patients invariably swallow their sputum and it may, therefore, be necessary, if tuberculosis is suspected, to look for rubencle bacilli in the stomach. The patient should be fasting and a tube introduced into the stomach. Sterile saline is injected and then withdrawn by a syringe.

Faeces. The bladder should first be emptied to avoid urine in the faecal specimen. In hospitals, a bedpan can be employed. This has usually been pasteurized in a bed pan washer. In private houses the collection of faeces may prove difficult. The methods available include the use of a chamber pot, or putting large quantities of lavatory paper in the bowl of the water closet to give a dry surface above the water. Another method is for the patient to defaecate into a plastic bag so arranged as to hang down into the lavatory bowl. It sometimes becomes necessary to use a rectal swab. A piece of faeces about the size of a large bean is enough for laboratory investigations. In cases of dysentery it is advisable to select mucus and blood stained portions for examination. The specimen should be transferred to a plastic screw-capped container. Usually the small spoon attached to the lid of the container is used.

Urine. The diagnosis of urinary tract infection is based on the number of organisms present in the urine. For this reason it is important that clean uncontaminated specimens are sent to the laboratory and that they are transported in such a way that any organisms that have been introduced at the time of collection are not allowed to multiply. In the case of males, a mid-stream specimen collected in a screw-capped sterile bottle is adequate. For females fundamentally the same method is used, the urine first passed being allowed to run away when the so-called clean catch specimen is collected in a screw-capped bottle with a wide neck. Because of the danger of the introduction of infection, chatheterization should be avoided.

In some patients the collection of clean specimens of urine may be difficult. In babies a special small plastic bag with an adhesive area may be attached to the perineum. Specimens obtained from the bags are often contaminated and if necessary urine may be obtained from babies by the technique of supra-public aspiration. This, in an infant, is a relatively simple procedure and produces an uncontaminated specimen.

However the specimen is obtained the method of transport to the laboratory is important. The specimen may be refrigerated and transported quickly. This method may not be practicable and borate bottles which maintain the urine in the condition in which it was passed for several hours may be used. Another possibility is the use of dip slides. These are commercially prepared plastic slides coated on both sides with media. They are dipped into the urine immediately after it has been passed and then transported to the laboratory in their own container. The slides are incubated and the amount of growth indicates whether or not infection is present.

Vagina and cervix uteri. If the lesions are present on the labia, specimens can be obtained by means of a swab, but if they are within the vagina or on the cervix, the patient must be placed in the lithotomy or left lateral position and a speculum employed to enable the specimen to be taken from the lesion. In puerperal infections, introduction of a swab into the vaginal cavity without the use of a speculum is adequate.

Cerebrospinal fluid. It is not necessary to describe the technique employed for obtaining specimens of cerebrospinal fluid, but it is advisable to point out that in view of the tragic consequences that may follow entry of pathogenic organisms into the spinal column, great care must be taken over the sterilization of the apparatus employed, in the preparation of the skin, and in the performance of the operation itself.

The fluid obtained should be delivered into a sterile bottle for examination and culture.

Blood. Blood may be required for culture or for ascertaining whether antibodies have made their appearance. For the former, it must be taken from a vein, usually one of those in the antecubital fossa. A 5 or 10 ml sterile syringe is necessary. The blood must be inoculated into liquid medium at the bedside and the mixture shaken to prevent the formation of a firm clot.

Blood for antibody examination is taken in the same way, but should be delivered, after removal of the needle, direct into a sterile tube or bottle. No anticoagulant such as citrate or oxalate must be present in the tube. This is a matter of some importance for anticoagulants are required when the blood is required for biochemical examination. For this reason, it is advisable for the nurse to ascertain what type of investigation is contemplated.

Purulent exudates. Pus is preferable to a swab, particularly if examination for anaerobic organism is required. It should be placed in a small bottle and delivered quickly to the laboratory.

Skin. Pus or other secretions can be picked up on wool swabs. But in some infections, it may first be necessary to remove crusts, etc. Scrapings of the skin may be required for the diagnosis of fungal infections.

Hair. For the diagnosis of ringworm, stumps of hairs should be selected for examination. Assistance in finding them may be obtained by the use of a Wood's lamp, since infected hairs tend to fluoresce in ultraviolet light.

Eye infections. A small wool swab placed in the inner canthus will usually suffice. An alternative method is to sample the same area with a sterile platinum loop and inoculate culture media at once.

Specimens from infections suspected to be due to viruses. The particular specimens required vary with the virus concerned, but on the whole, are not very different from those required for bacterial infections. Nevertheless, viruses are rather more susceptible than bacteria to physical influences such as drying and heat for which reason particular care should be taken that swabs for example, are placed at once in the special transport medium usually provided and that all the specimens are kept as cold as possible.

In all virus infections it is of considerable assistance if a specimen of blood be taken as early as possible in the illness and a second during convalescence, to ascertain whether antibodies for the virus suspected of causing the infection appear during the illness.

Food. In outbreaks of food infection or food poisoning any suspected articles of food, unopened cans or jars, etc., should be sought for. No attempt should be made to open such containers which should be sent direct to the laboratory. Scraps of food, etc., should be placed in sterile jars or other containers as soon as possible and kept cold.

THE MICRO-ORGANISMS RESPONSIBLE FOR DISEASE

In the five chapters that follow, each of the organisms that cause human diseases are described together with the signs and symptoms of the diseases and the sources from which they have probably come. A summary will also be given under the heading *Diagnosis*, of the methods that will probably be employed by the microbiologist to isolate and identify the infecting organism and determine its sensitivity to chemotherapeutic substances. The technical details of these procedures are purposely omitted. But it can undoubtedly, be of considerable assistance to everyone concerned, if the nurse has some idea of what investigations are likely to be carried out so that she can prepare the necessary apparatus and instruments. It may also be of value if she knows how long some of the investigations are likely to take and indeed, whether it is possible with the facilities available in the ordinary hospital laboratory, to make a bacteriological diagnosis at all.

The information given under *Treatment* is not meant to be complete or exhaustive. All that is included are the agents that actually deal with the organisms themselves. If no such agent is available, as is only too frequently the case in infections by viruses, the laconic statement, 'None' does not mean that it is impossible to help the patient at all. It merely means that that no drug has been discovered that can kill or check the organisms in any way.

The heading *Preventive measures*, is also restricted to those methods which are known to prevent infection by the particular organism concerned. And since most of these measures have already been discussed in some detail in the preceding chapters, they are merely summarized.

10

The cocci

The staphylococcus

Staphylococcus aureus

These are spherical particles about 0.001 mm in diameter.

Staphylococci cause infections of the skin such as furunculosis, *styes, boils, carbuncles, paronychia* and *impetigo,* infections of exposed tissues following *wounds, burns* and *scalds* and of deep tissues such as the tendon sheaths in *whitlows,* bones in *osteomyelitis* and the *lungs* following certain virus infections of which influenza is the most important. *Conjunctivitis, mastitis* and certain *skin infections* in new-born babies and *enterocolitis* following abdominal operations may also be due to this organism.

Certain strains can also form an *enterotoxin* if they are able to grow in foodstuffs such as meat dishes, and those containing milk in the form of custard, trifle, cake fillings and icings. When eaten, the toxin produces *acute diarrhoea* and *vomiting* from which recovery in about 24 hours is the rule.

About 50 per cent of normal human beings are nasal carriers and 25 per cent perineal carriers.

Diagnosis: The organisms can generally be seen by microscopic examination of the pus, or exudates from the lesions.

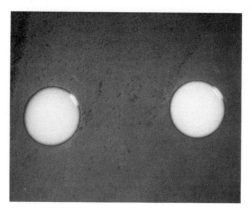

Fig. 10.1 Colonies of *Staphylococcus aureus.*

They produce dull yellow colonies on agar which clot citrated human plasma if they are mixed with it on a microscope slide. They are, therefore, said to be *coagulase positive.* Colonies of *Staph. albus* (a commensal) are white and *coagulase negative.* Different types of staphylococci are detected by *phage typing.*

Treatment: For pyogenic infections, penicillin for sensitive strains; penicillin resistant staphylococci may be treated with penicillinase resistant penicillins such as cloxacillin. For enterotoxic poisoning, none.

Preventive measures: For pyogenic infections, isolation of patients with infections; use of the no-touch technique when wounds are dressed or examined; wearing of gloves when babies or wounds must be handled (see p. 93). For enterotoxic poisoning, cleanliness in the kitchen and refrigeration of food, particularly when it contains milk or milk products.

The streptococci

Streptococci are about the same size as staphylococci but form chains.

They can be subdivided into three categories according to the way they behave when grown on agar containing blood.

1. *Haemolytic streptococci* produce haemolysis or dissolution of the red cells in the medium round the colonies.
2. *Streptococcus viridans* changes the red haemoglobin to a green compound round the colonies.

3. *Non-haemolytic streptococci* do not alter the blood in any way.

1. The haemolytic streptococcus

Streptococcus pyogenes

Although many varieties of streptococci can produce haemolysis, only those containing a certain carbohydrate which places them in Lancefield's Group A, are markedly pathogenic for human beings. Such organisms are frequently referred to as *Streptococcus pyogenes*.

The commonest form of infection produced by this organism is *acute tonsillitis* in which there is a whitish exudate on the tonsils with swelling of the cervical lymph glands, a sore throat and a high temperature. The infection may remain localized and soon subsides but occasionally it spreads up the eustachian tube to cause *otitis media* or *mastoiditis*.

Some strains produce exactly the same signs and symptoms but a bright red erythematous rash with circumoral pallor and a 'strawberry tongue' develop as well. The patient is then said to have *scarlet fever*. The additional signs are due to the formation by the organisms of the so-called erythrogenic toxin, but strange to say, they do not necessarily render the disease more severe or more infectious. Thus, scarlet fever is fundamentally the same disease as tonsillitis.

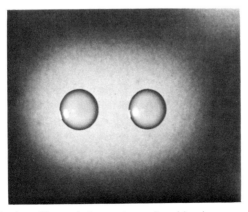

Fig. 10.2 Colonies of haemolytic streptococci on blood agar.

Complete and uninterrupted recovery usually occurs, but some patients may, after a silent period' of three weeks, become ill again with acute *rheumatic fever* or acute *nephritis*. Neither disease is due to the presence of the streptococci in the affected organs and their connection with the preceding streptococcal infection is still unexplained.

Haemolytic streptococci may also produce infection of *wounds, burns, scalds* and the placental site after delivery or abortion (*puerperal fever*). A third form of infection is *erysipelas* in which the organism invades the skin to produce a bright red patch with a slightly raised margin but without much tendency to suppuration. It occurs most frequently on the face. *Impetigo* is another skin infection that may be due to this organism.

Except for some cases of tonsillitis or scarlet fever which follow the drinking of unpasteurized milk from infected cows, all the infections mentioned above are due to organisms coming from human beings. They may be suffering from an infection but about 7 per cent of the population are symptomless throat carriers and about 1 per cent are nasal carriers. In hospitals, cross infection from other patients can occur.

Diagnosis: Chains of cocci in films made from pus, exudates, etc., can generally be seen and the organisms can be easily cultivated on blood agar.

Treatment: Benzyl penicillin or erythromycin.

Preventive measures: For tonsillitis and scarlet fever, nothing except isolation of cases. For wound and puerperal infections, similar measures as in a staphylococcal infections but carriers, if found, must be sent off duty.

2. Streptococcus viridans

This organism is a normal commensal in the human throat, but it may be associated with infection of the gums or tooth sockets and be forced into the blood stream during mastication or the extraction of teeth. The organisms quickly disappear from the blood but may very occasionally settle on the valves of the heart particularly if they are diseased, to cause *subacute bacterial endocarditis*. This is the most important pathogenic activity of this organism.

Diagnosis: Blood culture, in subacute bacterial endocarditis, is the method of diagnosis

Treatment: Massive doses of penicillin.

Preventive measures: Prophylactic doses of antibiotics when teeth are extracted.

3. The non-haemolytic streptococci

Although streptococci coming within this category are present in the throat and nose of all human beings and quite frequently in the faeces as well, they seldom cause serious infections. The exceptions are the different varieties of anaerobic streptococci found in the vagina, which may cause a form of *puerperal fever* after delivery, and the enterococci which cause urinary tract infection and occasionally subacute bacterial endocarditis.

The pneumococcus

Diplococcus pneumoniae

This organism is about the same size as a staphylococcus but is generally found in pairs, and is surrounded by a well-marked capsule.

The most important disease produced by this organism is *pneumonia.* The onset is usually sudden with fever, pain in the

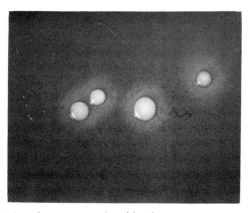

Fig. 10.3 Colonies of pneumococci on blood agar.

chest and cough with rusty, i.e. blood-stained, sputum. The illness proceeds rapidly and if untreated, death may occur in about a week in a high proportion of cases. This organism may also cause *secondary infection* in the respiratory tract following a virus infection such as a cold, measles or influenza. This in turn may bring about *otitis media* and, in the more severe cases, *mastoiditis*. Meningitis is an important disease which may be caused by the pneumococcus and peritonitis and, occasionally, infection of wounds may also be caused by this organism. Many normal persons are symptomless throat carriers.

Diagnosis: The organism can be seen in films of the sputum in pneumonia, the cerebrospinal fluid in meningitis and in the pus from cases of otitis media. It can also be easily cultivated on blood agar.

Treatment: Penicillin.

Preventive measures: None.

The meningococcus

Neisseria meningitidis

This organism is about the same size as a staphylococcus but is generally seen in pairs.

It is responsible for many cases of meningitis or *cerebrospinal fever*. This disease occurs as a sporadic infection in children or in small epidemics amongst young adults, particularly recruits in the armed forces. The organism invades the blood stream from the nose and so reaches the meninges to cause purulent meningitis. The patient is extremely ill with fever, headache and signs of meningeal irritation. A petechial or purpuric rash may also develop on the first or second day. Death usually occurs in the absence of treatment.

The organism may be derived from other cases but more often from a symptomless carrier. Many normal persons have this organism in the nose or throat.

Diagnosis: Microscopic examination of stained films from the cerebrospinal fluid shows the presence of polymorphonuclear leucocytes, many of which contain pairs of Gram-negative cocci. They will grow if the fluid is added to glucose broth and incubated in an atmosphere of carbon dioxide.

Treatment: Sulphonamides and penicillin.
Preventive measures: None, other than avoidance of over-crowding.

The gonococcus

Neisseria gonorrhoea

This organism is very similar to the meningococcus.

It produces gonorrhoea, a venereal infection of the urethra which may spread to the seminal vesicles, prostate, epididymis and testicles in the male, or Bartholin's glands, the fallopian tubes and ovaries in the female. Metastic *infection of joints* sometimes occurs. When present in the birth canal at the time of delivery, the organisms may reach the eyes of the child and produce an acute purulent conjunctivitis known as *ophthalmia neonatorum*. A third form of infection is *vulvo-vaginitis* in female children.

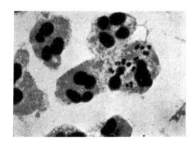

Fig. 10.4 Gonococci in pus from the urethra.

Diagnosis: The characteristic Gram-negative diplococci can be seen in the cells of the exudate from the urethra or the cervix in females but in chronic cases culture may be necessary. Since the organisms may not survive drying or exposure to oxygen, it is advisable to inoculate the culture medium in the clinic or immerse swabs impregnated with the pus in a special 'holding medium' for transport to the laboratory. Media containing blood or blood heated until it has become the colour of chocolate, are required for culture and the plates must be incubated in an atmosphere containing 10–20 per cent carbon dioxide.

Treatment: Penicillin, but large doses may be necessary because some strains are partially resistant. Penicillinase producing gonococci are becoming more common and are treated with spectinomycin.

Preventive measures: For gonorrhoea, none other than avoidance of sexual promiscuity. For ophthalmia neonatorum, instillation of penicillin into the eyes of babies born of infected mothers.

11

The bacilli and vibrios

A great many organisms must be considered in this chapter. They vary greatly in appearance, the sources from which they come, the type of disease they produce and the organs most likely to be infected. All can, however, be placed in one or other of six well marked groups.

A. BACILLI ASSOCIATED WITH THE RESPIRATORY TRACT

1. The diphtheria bacillus

Corynebacterium diphtheriae

This organism is about 0.003 mm long, not motile and unable to produce spores, capsules or flagella. Circular bodies at one or both ends can be stained an intense black by special stains (Neisser or Albert).

It causes *diphtheria* after an incubation period of 2–4 days. A 'false membrane' develops consisting of fibrin and necrotic cells in which are large numbers of the bacilli. It is usually situated on the tonsils and fauces but it may extend into the nose or to the larynx and into the trachea. The organism may also infect *wounds*, the *vulva* and *conjunctiva* in populations living under conditions of extreme poverty as in the Near and Far East.

173

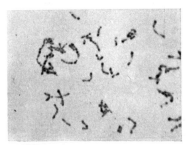

Fig. 11.1 Diphtheria bacilli.

Due to the formation of a powerful exotoxin by the organisms, there is marked toxaemia and in some cases, paralysis of the palate and muscles of accommodation together with degeneration of the myocardium. This may be sufficiently severe to cause death. But death may also result from suffocation if the false membrane becomes so extensive that it blocks the larynx or trachea.

Symptomless nose or throat carriers are fairly common in places where the disease is endemic but are very rare indeed where the disease has disappeared following widespread immunization.

Diagnosis: The diagnosis of diphtheria must generally be made clinically. It is sometimes possible to diagnose the disease by microscopic examination of smears from the false membrane but the organism grows in less than 24 hours on a Loeffler slope (coagulated ox serum) or on special media containing tellurite.

Treatment: Antitoxic serum, with penicillin or erythromycin.

Preventive measures: Prophylactic immunization with toxoid in infancy, with booster doses on going to school, at the age of 10–11 and again when leaving school.

Isolation of cases, administration of erythromycin to carriers.

2. Haemophilus

Haemophilus influenzae

This is a minute coccobacillus about 0.002 mm long and without spores or flagella.

Despite its name, this organism does not cause influenza but may be responsible for infections in the nasal sinuses and for some cases of *bronchitis*. Certain capsulated strains cause a severe variety of *meningitis* in children.

This organism can be found in almost all normal throats.

Diagnosis: In meningitis, microscopic examination of the cerebrospinal fluid will show that large numbers of tiny coccobacilli as well as long thread-like forms are present. Special media are required to isolate it because it requires vitamins and other growth-promoting substances to a much greater extent than other organisms.

Treatment: Chloramphenicol or ampicillin for meningitis, tetracycline, ampicillin or cotrimoxazole for bronchitis.

Preventive measures: None.

3. The whooping cough bacillus

Bordetella pertusis

This organism is a tiny coccobacillus only 0.001 to 0.002 mm in length. No spores, flagella or capsules are produced.

It is the causative agent of *whooping cough*. The incubation period is 10 to 14 days. The child then becomes ill with catarrhal symptoms in the throat accompanied by a cough. At first, the cough does not seem to be unusual but after a day or two paroxysms of whooping begin. These start with a long inspiration, then a series of short expiratory barks during which no air enters the chest and the child appears to be suffocating. The condition is relieved suddenly by a long inspiration or whoop. Vomiting is common after such a paroxysm.

Older children usually recover but before the first birthday, whooping cough is an important cause of death, due largely to complications such as collapse of a lung, bronchopneumonia and encephalopathy.

Diagnosis: Two methods may be used. Cough plates consisting of petri dishes containing the special medium necessary (Bordet Gengou medium) are held in front of and slightly below the level of the mouth during the paroxysms. Characteristic colonies resembling globules of mercury appear after incubation for two or more days.

Alternatively, secretions may be obtained from the postnasal space, using a thin wire swab thrust through the nostrils, or a bent swab introduced by way of the fauces, and the organism isolated on the same medium as that used for the cough plates.

Treatment: Antibiotics would appear to have little value but ampicillin is probably the most useful.

Preventive measures: Prophylactic immunization with killed organisms undoubtedly protects against the disease but there is some risk that neurological complications may occur as a result of their administration. However there is a definite risk of death from the disease amongst un-immunized children, so immunization is still recommended.

4. Klebsiella

Klebsiella pneumoniae: Klebsiella aerogenes

These are comparatively short bacilli surrounded by a large capsule.

Under normal circumstances *Klebsiella pneumoniae* is a commensal in the throat of human beings and may occasionally cause *pneumonia*. However *Klebsiella aerogenes* has become important in recent years as a cause of serious infection in debilitated or immunosuppressed patients in hospitals.

Diagnosis. The organisms grow rapidly on solid medium and form very large mucoid colonies.

Treatment: Difficult, a combination of antibiotics may be necessary.

Preventive measures: None for *Klebsiella pneumonia.* Hospital infection preventive measures for *Klebsiella aerogenes* infections.

5. Legionnaire's disease bacillus

Legionella pneumophila

This small Gram-negative bacillus has only recently been described. It is a fastidious organism widely distributed in nature and is the causative agent of bronchopneumonia. Associated with this may be mental confusion and impaired renal function. The name arises because the first clearly recorded outbreak of the disease was in a group of Legionnaires attending a congress. The source of the organism is often contaminated water such as may be found in air conditioning systems and shower heads.

Diagnosis: Usually made by showing a rise in antibody titre.

Treatment: Erythromycin.

Preventive measures: Ensure that reservoirs of water particularly those which may form an aerosol are kept clean and periodically disinfected.

B. BACILLI ASSOCIATED WITH THE INTESTINAL CANAL

The organisms in this group may be found in the intestinal tract as commensals or pathogens but some may cause infection in other parts of the body.

1. The coliform bacillus

Escherichia coli

These are all short rods (0.004–0.005 mm long) without capsules or spores. They possess flagella and are therefore motile. All are Gram-negative.

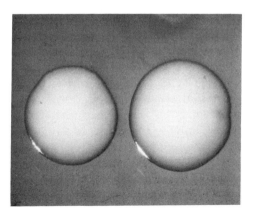

Fig. 11.2 Colonies of coliform bacilli.

Such organisms are invariably present in the intestinal canal of human beings as commensals but can cause *peritonitis* if the intestinal contents get into the peritoneal cavity. They may also cause *cystitis* and *pyelonephritis*. Certain strains cause gastro-enteritis in young children. It has also been found recently that these organisms are capable of producing *bacteraemic* shock as a result of their sudden invasion of the blood stream.

Diagnosis: The bacilli can be seen in films of the pus or urine. They grow easily and ferment the sugar lactose, whereas the other gastro-intestinal bacilli with which they might be confused, are unable to do so. Agglutination tests are necessary to identify the special types responsible for gastro-enteritis.

Treatment: Ampicillin, trimethoprim-sulphonamide.

Preventive measures: For infections of the peritoneum none. For gastro-enteritis in children, preliminary isolation of all admittances, to ascertain whether or not they have diarrhoea. Sterilization of feeding bottles, teats and the avoidance of transfer or the organism to the baby's mouth by way of the fingers of the nurse.

2. The typhoid and paratyphoid bacilli

Salmonella typhi; Salmonella paratyphi A; Salmonella paratyphi B; Salmonella paratyphi C

These organisms closely resemble the coliform bacilli in appearance but some do not possess flagella. None of them can ferment the sugar lactose whereas the coliform bacilli are able to do so.

They reach the patient in food, water or milk and invade the lymphatics in the Peyer's patches of the small intestine. After an incubation period of about 12 days, they reach the blood stream. The patient soon becomes extremely ill with the steadily mounting fever and the rose spots on the skin characteristic of *typhoid* or *paratyphoid fever*, collectively known as *enteric*. Metastatic abscesses may occur in almost any part of the body. Of much greater importance, however, is the weakening of the intestinal wall at the Peyer's patches for this may lead to perforation into the peritoneal cavity or haemorrhage from ruptured vessels in the wall of the gut. The illness may last 3 or more weeks; recovery is always slow and relapses are common.

The organisms are invariably derived from the urine or faeces of another human being who may be a patient suffering from the disease, a convalescent carrier or a permanent carrier. Some carriers may have had the disease in so mild a form that they are unaware they have had it.

Diagnosis: The organisms can generally be isolated by blood culture during the first two weeks of the disease. They can also be isolated from the faeces at the same time and often for long periods during convalescence. The particular variety of organism responsible for the infection can only be determined by agglutination tests.

After the fourteenth day, it is frequently possible to diagnose the disease by the *Widal test*. This depends on the fact that antibodies make their appearance in the circulating blood so that the serum of the patient agglutinates or clumps a culture of the organisms.

Treatment: Chloramphenicol or ampicillin.

Preventive measures: Care in the disposal of faeces, eradication of flies, screening of larders, filtration or chlorination of water supplies, washing of hands after defaecation. Prophylactic immunization with T.A.B. vaccine. Barrier nursing of cases in hospitals. Control of known carriers.

3. The food infection bacilli

Salmonella typhi-murium, etc.

These organisms also resemble the coliform bacilli but cannot ferment the sugar lactose.

There are many different species of *Salmonella* but that which is most frequently responsible for food infection is *Salmonella typhimurium*. Whatever the species, the organism always reaches human beings in food and produces *food infection* or *food poisoning* as it is frequently, but incorrectly, called. The incubation period is usually about 24 hours following which there is acute diarrhoea and vomiting. This seldom lasts for more than 24–48 hours when recovery sets in.

Infections of this type are still very common and although recovery soon occurs when the patient is healthy, an illness of this nature may be very serious when the patient is already debilitated by some other disease. The prevention of the disease amongst hospital patients is therefore a matter of considerable importance in which the nurse can play an important part.

The food responsible is usually meat from an infected animal which has been processed in such a way that the organisms have not been killed. Eggs from infected fowls or ducks may also convey the organisms. They may also come from a human case or carrier, being conveyed on the hands to food which is consumed without further cooking. Flies may also convey the organisms from the faeces to food.

Diagnosis: Specimens of vomit and faeces should be taken and cultures of the organisms obtained. They must then be identified by agglutination reactions. Attempts must also be made to isolate the organism from food or drink suspected of being the cause.

Treatment: Only required when the infection is severe and the patient is debilitated or dehydrated when neomycin, tetracyclines, or the insoluble sulphonamides may be used.

Preventive measures: Care in the selection of animals for slaughtering, the maintenance of high standards of cleanliness in food processing factories and adequate methods for sterilization of foods that are preserved by canning. Cooking at temperatures high enough to ensure killing of the organisms and preservation of foods in a refrigerator after cooking.

Provision of washing facilities in restaurants, the avoidance of handling of such foods as sandwiches that are eaten without cooking, thorough washing of vegetables and fruits, and the elimination of flies.

4. The dysentery bacilli

Shigella sonnei; Shigella flexneri; Shigella shigae

These organisms also resemble the coliform bacilli but have no flagella and do not ferment lactose. Several species are known. The most widely prevalent organism in Western countries is *Shigella sonnei*. In the East, *Shigella flexneri* or *Shigella shigae* are more usual.

They are human organisms, present in the faeces of both

carriers and cases and therefore easily transmissible from person to person to produce *dysentery*. After an incubation period of about 48 hours, there occurs acute vomiting, headache, pyrexia and the frequent passage of small stools. These are faecal at first but in time consist of mucus and blood. In the later stages of the more severe cases, pure blood may be passed.

Recovery generally occurs in infections by *Shigella sonnei* after an acute stage lasting several days, but in the more severe forms due to other species the symptoms become more marked and death may eventually occur. Carriers of dysentery bacilli are common in places where the disease is prevalent.

Outbreaks of dysentery are comparatively common in institutions such as asylums where the personal habits of some patients may be lax, or in camps where faeces must be deposited in buckets or latrines. Dysentery is also a very common disease in hot countries with defective sanitation.

Diagnosis: The stools usually contain mucus and this should be selected for examination. Since dysentery may also be due to a protozoon called *Entamoeba histolytica* it is first necessary to ascertain by microscopical examination whether or not this organism is present. If it is not, and red blood cells and pus cells can be seen it is probable that one or other of the dysentery bacilli is responsible. This may be confirmed by culture, isolation of the organisms, and their identification by agglutination reactions.

Treatment: Unnecessary in most infections by *Sh. sonnei.* In the more severe forms, neomycin, tetracyclines, or the insoluble sulphonamides may be used.

Preventive measures: Care in the disposal of faeces. Eradication of flies. Hand washing after defaecation.

5. Proteus

Proteus vulgaris, Proteus mirabilis, Proteus morgani, Proteus rettgeri

These organisms grow in the form of bacilli which vary from very long to very short. No spores are produced, but the organisms possess large numbers of flagella and are highly motile.

These organisms are comparatively common in decomposing animal matter, in soil and in dust. But they can also survive in the alimentary canal as commensals so that they may also be present in the faeces of human beings. It is from such sources that infections are acquired. They may reach the urinary tract to cause *pyelonephritis* or *cystitis* particularly when micturition is disturbed. They can also act as secondary invaders when *wounds* or *burns* are infected by other organisms. Such organisms can also produce *bacteraemic shock.*

Diagnosis: Although this organism can be easily seen, it is not sufficiently characteristic in appearance for microscopic examination of pus, urine, etc., to be employed for diagnosis. This depends on the fact that instead of growing, like most organisms, in the form of separate or distinctive colonies on solid medium, it forms a thin continuous sheet of growth over its surface. A useful confirmatory test is the ability of this organism to attack urea with the formation of ammonia. This can be detected by using suitable media.

Treatment: Ampicillin trimethoprim-sulphonamide, nitrofurantoin for urinary infections.

Preventive measures: None.

6. Pseudomonas

Pseudomonas aeruginosa

This organism is a rather slender, somewhat pointed rod about 0.003 mm in length and is motile because of flagella at each end.

It produces infection of *wounds*, particularly those resulting from accidents: *burns* and *scalds* may likewise be infected. Although it is seldom the cause of *post-operative infection*, it may do so. The *lungs* too may become infected particularly in the old or debilitated. *Eyes* have also become infected following operations for cataract. This organism is one of those responsible for acute *bacteraemic shock* caused by sudden flooding of the blood stream by organisms from a septic focus.

This organism is frequently present in moist situations such as faeces and water supplies. Even that of hospitals may contain it. The organism may directly reach susceptible tissues

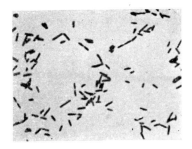

Fig. 11.3 Microscopic appearance of *Pseudomonas aeruginosa*.

from such sources but it can also cause cross infection as well. Since it can multiply in the presence of very little nutrient material it may be found in supposedly sterile water to cause wound infection or in that of humidifiers to bring about pneumonia. It is also more resistant than most organisms to antiseptics so that it may be present alive in solutions of antiseptics such as cetrimide.

Diagnosis: This organism cannot be identified by microscopic examination but when cultivated, the medium acquires a green or blue tint in the neighbourhood of the organism.

Treatment: Gentamicin, carbenicillin, azlocillin.

Preventive measures: The no-touch technique for dressings. Sterilization of urinals and humidifier bottles. Care in the use of antiseptics.

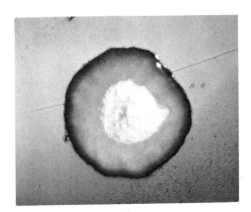

Fig. 11.4 Colony of *Pseudomonas aeruginosa*.

7. Bacteroides

Fusiform bacilli

This organism is a cigar shaped rod which, unlike those described above, can only multiply in the absence of oxygen.

Common in the mouth and intestinal tract its importance in causing infection has only recently been appreciated. In association with the Vincent's angina spirochaete it can cause a severe infection in the mouth. However, it can also cause serious infections in many other parts of the body, particularly wound infections.

Diagnosis: These organisms may be difficult to isolate. Strictly anaerobic conditions are required for culture and rapid transport to the laboratory or the use of transport media are also necessary.

Treatment: Metronidazole

Preventive measures: Prophylactic antibiotics at the time of operation.

C. ACID FAST BACILLI

These organisms are thin rods that may be slightly curved. Using the Ziehl Neelsen method of staining they are 'acid fast' and are therefore red whereas all other organisms are blue. No spores, capsules or flagella are formed.

1. The tubercle bacillus

Mycobacterium tuberculosis

The tubercle bacillus is a thin rod which may be slightly curved. No spores, capsules or flagella are formed.

The tubercle bacillus can infect almost any tissue and any organ to produce the characteristic signs and symptoms of *tuberculosis*. These are the consequences of the slow but inexorable spread of the disease process through the tissues and the injury to any important structures that may lie in its path. This inevitably causes local pain, swelling and disability with more general symptoms such as pyrexia, night sweats, loss of weight and appetite with, as the disease advances, increasing cachexia and finally death. Wherever the focus of infection is situated, the disease is always chronic but in certain forms such as *tuberculous meningitis* and *miliary tuberculosis* in which the organism reaches the meninges or blood stream respectively, the symptoms become suddenly worse and death soon occurs.

In communities in which tuberculosis of the lungs is common, there is reason to believe that subclinical infection by the tubercle bacillus is a common event during childhood. As a result of inhalation of the organisms, a strictly localized area of infection develops in one lung. This soon heals leaving an area of fibrosis in the lung which is called the Ghon focus.

As a result of such a subclinical infection or, indeed, clinically obvious infection as well, the individual becomes *allergic* to tuberculin—a protein formed by the organism. If, then, tuberculin is injected into his skin a reaction consisting of oedema and erythema is produced. Such an individual is said to be Mantoux positive, and is more likely to escape tuberculosis in adult life than those who have escaped infection altogether and are lMantoux negative. Largely because of the increasing rarity of the disease in advanced communities, immunity may not be acquired in this way. Migrants from such communities to those where the disease is still common are obviously at a disadvantage and may become infected soon after their arrival.

The great majority of infections are caused by the so-called human type of the organism. But a variant known as the bovine type may cause infection in cows and is excreted in the milk. This may be responsible for human infections principally of the abdominal lymph glands and of joints. This too is becoming unusual.

Diagnosis: Whenever possible, an attempt must be made to ascertain that the organisms are present. In pulmonary tuberculosis, the sputum, preferably the first expectoration of the morning, is examined but with children who swallow the sputum it may be necessary to resort to stomach washings for this purpose. In tuberculosis of the urinary tract the organism is generally present in the urine. Three early morning specimens should be obtained and the sediment allowed to settle. Films are made from the sediment, stained and examined microscopically. In tuberculous meningitis, cerebrospinal fluid must

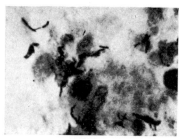

Fig. 11.5 Tubercle bacilli in sputum.

be obtained and the organism searched for in the clot which usually forms after collection. In other forms of the disease, the organisms can generally be seen in pus, aspirated fluid or biopsies obtained from the infected area.

The organisms can be isolated on special media made from egg yolk but growth is so slow that a delay of 4 to 6 weeks is inevitable. But once isolated, its identity can be confirmed and its sensitivity to antibiotics determined.

Treatment: Streptomycin, rifampicin, ethambutol, para-aminosalicylic acid, isoniazid, thioacetazone.

Preventive measures: Detection and isolation of all cases of pulmonary tuberculosis with treatment until cured and education in the disposal of sputum. If in general hospitals they should be barrier nursed. Betterment of nutrition and living conditions in underdeveloped countries, administration of B.C.G. and pasteurization of milk.

2. The leprosy bacillus

Mycobacterium leprae

This organism closely resembles the tubercle bacillus. It is also acid fast.

It is responsible for *leprosy*, an extremely chronic disease usually acquired as a result of prolonged close contact with other cases. It occurs in two forms—nodular and anaesthetic. The former tends to attack the face and nasal mucous membranes, but other areas of skin may also be involved. The lesions produce serious changes in the facial appearance and the voice, while nodules and masses may appear on the limbs.

In the anaesthetic form, maculae appear on the skin with erythema and alterations in its pigmentation. These areas may spread and become anaesthetic so that in the final stage of the disease there may be dry parchment-like skin with perforating ulcers or actual loss of limbs or parts of limbs from injuries sustained by the anaesthetic areas.

Diagnosis: It is not possible to cultivate the organisms but acid-fast bacilli may be seen in the nasal secretions, in the cells from scrapings of the nasal mucous membrane or in excised pieces of skin from infected areas.

Treatment: Sulphones.

Preventive measures: Segregation of lepers into special hospitals. Improvement in living conditions.

D. SPORE BEARING BACILLI

The four organisms in this group all produce spores that are extremely resistant to heat and antiseptics.

1. The tetanus bacillus

Clostridium tetani

This organism is a comparatively slender bacillus with flagella that render it highly motile. It produces a spherical spore at one end of the bacillus. It is wider than the bacillus itself so that the two together resemble a drumstick. A second peculiarity is that this organism will only grow in the complete absence of oxygen and a third, is its ability to produce an extremely powerful exotoxin.

It is responsible for the fortunately rare disease, *tetanus*. This usually follows a traumatic wound, but it occasionally occurs after clean operations. In backward countries where little regard is paid to sterility it may occur in the mother following an abortion or full term delivery or as an infection of the cord in new-born children.

The symptoms are almost all due to the formation of a specific exotoxin by the organisms growing in the wound. This may produce local tetanus in which there is stiffness and rigidity in the neighbouring muscles. But in the more severe cases, the rigidity becomes so widespread that the patient cannot even open his mouth and because of this, the disease was once known as lockjaw. Convulsions or spasms may also occur in which practically every muscle in the body contracts so strongly that there is arching of the back or opisthotonus. The wound itself may appear to be quite clean and there are no symptoms usually associated with infection.

This organism survives and probably multiplies in soil. It is also frequently found in the intestinal canal of animals. As a general rule, it is not the bacilli themselves that get into wounds. It is the spores. In most wounds, they cannot germinate because sufficient oxygen is present in the tissues to prevent it. But if there is local necrosis and anoxaemia, germination can then take place and the bacilli formed are then able to multiply and produce the toxin.

Diagnosis: So few organisms are generally present in the wound that it may be impossible to see or cultivate them.

Treatment: Antitoxic serum is of doubtful value. General measures such as relaxants.

Preventive measures: At operations, absolute sterility of all instruments, dressings, etc. Early cleansing of traumatic wounds, removal of all dead or dying tissue (débridement) and foreign bodies, and prophylactic penicillin.

Toxoid immunization in infancy with booster doses after any injury likely to be followed by the disease. But when there is no history of prior immunization, and the wound is severe, human globulin from immunized persons can be employed as a prophylactic.

2. The gas gangrene bacilli

Clostridium perfringens (welchii) Clostridium oedematiens, Clostridium septicum

These organisms are all comparatively large and form oat-shaped spores in the body of the bacillus, never at the end.

They are the cause of *gas gangrene*, an extremely severe infection of wounds and, very rarely, the placental site. The wound soon becomes discoloured with an abundant blood-stained exudate in which there may be bubbles of gas. The muscles below become dark and friable with gas in and around them. The symptoms, most of which are due to exotoxins produced by the organisms, comprise a high temperature, increased pulse rate, profound toxaemia and ultimately, death.

Like the tetanus bacillus, these organisms can only multiply in the absence of oxygen and form powerful exotoxins. Their sources and the train of events that lead to the development of infection are also similar.

Some strains of *Cl. perfringens* can cause a form of *food infection* if they are able to multiply in the food before it is eaten. The food in question is usually a stew which has been kept warm for several hours.

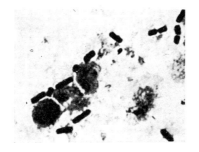

Fig. 11.6 Gas gangrene bacilli in the exudate from a wound.

Diagnosis: Comparatively large Gram-positive bacilli can generally be seen in films made from the exudate. The organisms grow rapidly in Robertson's meat medium (broth containing pieces of meat) or on solid medium, provided it is incubated anaerobically.

Treatment: Penicillin and antitoxic serum.

Preventive measures: Early débridement of wounds, sterility of instruments and dressings and prophylactic penicillin. Antitoxic serum is of doubtful value.

3. The botulism bacillus

Clostridium botulinum

This organism resembles those responsible for gas gangrene. Spores are formed within the body of the bacillus.

The disease, *botulism,* caused by this organism, is not due to multiplication of the organisms in the body of the patient, but to the absorption from the alimentary canal of toxins they have formed as a result of growth in food before it is eaten. Such symptoms appear within a few hours of the meal and are largely due to the action of the toxin on the cranial nerves. They comprise diplopia and paralysis of the muscles of accommodation, inability to swallow or speak and paralysis of the diaphragm. Death is the usual ending with the patient fully conscious to the last.

The spores of this organism generally come from soil, and get into food. If it is eaten at once, before they can germinate, the disease cannot follow its consumption. But if the food is canned, bottled or pickled, conditions are created that favour the germination of the spcres, growth of the organism and production of the toxin. For no very clear reason, this occurs so seldom that botulism is an extremely rare disease.

Diagnosis: It is not usually possible to isolate the organism from the patient, but food which may have been the cause of the condition must be kept and sent to the laboratory where the organisms can generally be isolated by growth in Robertson's meat medium.

Treatment: Administration of botulinus antitoxin.

Preventive measures: Care over the cleanliness of all utensils employed for the preparation of food that is to be preserved. Sufficiently high temperatures in canning or bottling

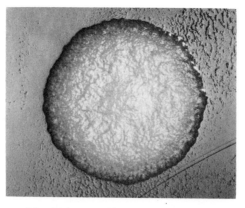

Fig. 11.7 Colony of *B. cereus* resembling that of the anthrax bacillus.

to ensure killing the spores. Storage of cans or bottles at low temperatures to prevent germination of the spores.

4. The bacillus of pseudo-membranous colitis

Clostridium difficile

The clinical importance of this *clostridium* has only recently been appreciated. After the administration of a number of antibiotics, particularly clindamycin, *Clostridium difficile* may be found in large numbers in the bowel and may cause a severe inflammation known as pseudo-membranous colitis.

Diagnosis: Demonstration of toxin in the faeces. Isolation of the organism. Biopsy of the mucosa.

Treatment: Stop antibiotic. Administer vancomycin.

Preventive measures: Care in the use of antibiotics particularly following bowel surgery. Prevention of spread of the organism in hospital wards.

4. The anthrax bacillus

Bacillus anthracis

This is a large square-ended bacillus growing in chains. Spores are formed in the centre of the organism. It does not possess flagella but may have a capsule.

This organism is different in a number of respects from those described above. It can for example, grow in the presence of oxygen.

Under normal circumstances, it is not a human organism. It produces *anthrax*, a generalized and invariably fatal infection of cattle and sheep. But if the organisms get into cuts or scratches on the skin of human beings, they produce a *malignant pustule*, an ulcer with a black necrotic base, raised edges and redness and oedema in the surrounding skin. This may progress to produce a generalized infection. A second form of the disease is *wool sorter's pneumonia* which follows inhalation of the spores from the wool or hides of infected animals.

Diagnosis: The large Gram-positive bacilli can be seen in smears from the infected areas and can be cultivated easily.

Treatment: Penicillin.

Preventive measures: Immediate slaughter and deep burial of all infected animals. Precautions in wool processing and leather factories to prevent inhalation of the spores.

E. BACILLI DERIVED FROM INFECTED ANIMALS

1. The plague bacillus

Yersinia pestis

This organism is a short, rather fat bacillus about 0.002 mm in length and without spores, flagella or capsules.

It is the causative agent of *plague.* In the commonest form of the disease usually referred to as *bubonic plague*, the glands in the groin and less often those in the axilla or neck become enlarged and intensely painful, while the patient is extremely ill and death may occur in only a few days. In the *septicaemic* and *pneumonic* forms the infection is more generalized and the death rate may be as high as 100 per cent.

The plague bacillus is fundamentally a pathogen of rats and other rodents producing a disease somewhat resembling bubonic plague in human beings. The organisms are transmitted from animal to animal by rat fleas and it is as a result of a bite by an infected flea that human beings acquire the disease.

Although human cases of the disease occur in India, and other countries in the East, in which case the organisms have generally come from rats, it is worthy of note that outbreaks of the disease have occurred in Mongolia from tar tarbaraghs and more recently in the western United States where the animals involved were ground squirrels.

Diagnosis: Examination of fluid from the inflamed gland or the sputum in pneumonic cases, may reveal the presence of the typical oval organisms, whose identity can be confirmed by culture or by injection into rats or guinea pigs. These animals soon die with the organisms present in large numbers in the enlarged glands and spleen.

Treatment: Tetracyclines.

Preventive measures. Extermination of rats. Improvement in living conditions. Prophylactic immunization with vaccine. Spraying of dwellings with insecticides.

2. The brucellosis bacilli

Brucella abortus; Brucella melitensis; Brucella suis

All three species grow in the form of minute coccobacilli without flagella, capsules or spores.

They produce *brucellosis* or *undulant fever* which is chiefly characterized by the fact that the patient has long spells of pyrexia without signs of local infection anywhere. Such spells may occur again and again for a period of several years.

The organisms are invariably acquired from cattle, pigs or goats. They are natural pathogens of these animals, being responsible for the disease known as *contagious abortion*. Those in contact with infected animals, that is, farmers, workers in slaughter-houses and veterinarians may, therefore, be infected directly. The organisms may, however, invade the udder and so reach the milk. Consumption of unpasteurized milk is an alternative method of acquiring the disease.

Diagnosis: The most satisfactory method is to isolate the organism by blood culture but failure to do so is common and the organisms may take a month to grow. Diagnosis frequently depends on showing that antibodies have made their appearance in the circulating blood. They can be detected by their ability to agglutinate a culture of the organisms.

Treatment: Combined therapy with tetracyclines and streptomycin.

Preventive measures: Eradication of the disease in dairy herds by immunization and slaughter of infected animals. Improvements in hygiene of cattle sheds. Pasteurization of milk.

F. VIBRIOS

The cholera vibrio

Vibrio cholerae

This organism grows in the form of short curved rods. It is motile, with a flagellum at each end.

Cholera is an infection of the intestinal tract. The incubation

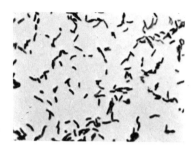

Fig. 11.8 Cholera vibrios.

period is only 6–24 hours and the onset is sudden with vomiting and the passage at short intervals of the characteristic rice water stools. This leads to loss of electrolytes and intense dehydration which is primarily the cause of death. There is also severe thirst, with suppressior of urine and muscular cramps. The organism may come from other cases of the disease, patients with only mild diarrhoea or from carriers and is spread from person to person by faecal contamination of food or water. Poor hygiene and sanitation accordingly play an important part in its dissemination and it is for this reason that the disease tends to be common in underdeveloped communities. Nevertheless, many such countries had been free of the disease for many years, but in 1970, the disease reached Africa, southern Europe and many countries in Asia to produce quite severe epidemics. Sporadic cases of the disease, usually developing in individuals from such places have also occurred in northern Europe and Australia.

Diagnosis: Microscopic examination of the stools may alone suffice, for the vibrios are present in enormous numbers. Culture should also be made and this establishes the diagnosis overnight.

Treatment: Saline given intravenously to relieve dehydration and replace electrolytes. Tetracycline.

Preventive measures: Isolation of the patients. Safe disposal of excreta. Eradication of flies. Chlorination of water supplies. Prophylactic immunization with vaccines.

Vibrio parahaemolyticus

This is a marine vibrio which causes a form of food poisoning associated with eating shellfish.

CAMPYLOBACTERS

Campylobacter jejuni; Campylobacter coli.

The bacteria are curved like the vibrios and used to be classified with them. They are the causative agents of a form of food poisoning. The source of the infection is often milk or intensively reared chickens.

Diagnosis: Isolation of the organism from faeces using special media at 43°C and incubated with a reduced oxygen tension.

Treatment: Usually none necessary; erythromycin may be given.

Prevention: Pasteurisation of milk. Care in the preparation and storage of food.

12

The spirochaetes

The spirochaetes are fundamentally long thin threads wound in the form of spirals. The number of convolutions varies from species to species. Six diseases may be caused by them.

1. The syphilis spirochaete

Treponema pallidum

This organism is a very long thin thread wound in the form of a spiral whose length is about 0.01 to 0.015 mm. It is actively motile.

It is responsible for the venereal disease, *syphilis*. The first sign is the appearance, after an incubation period of three to four weeks, of a small hard papule which is red in colour situated on the penis in males and the labia in females. It rapidly ulcerates to produce the *Primary Chancre* which eventually heals, even when untreated.

The *Secondary Stage* of the disease follows in five to twelve weeks in which the spirochaetes become widely disseminated throughout the body to produce sore throat, rashes, fever, loss of hair and various pathological lesions such as patches on mucous membranes, condylomata and swelling of the lymph glands.

196

These signs and symptoms eventually disappear and the patient may think that he has recovered completely. But after an interval, which may be as short as two years, but can be ten or more years, one or other manifestation of *Tertiary Syphilis* appears. These comprise localized areas of chronic inflammation called gummata, lesions in the skin, meningitis, disturbances of the cranial nerves to produce the Argyll Robertson pupil or of the central nervous system resulting in paralyses of the limbs or cranial nerves, tabes dorsalis and general paralysis of the insane.

Syphilis may also be acquired by the foetus from an infected mother. This usually leads to miscarriage, but if the child is born alive, it may have *congenital syphilis.* This involves changes in the eyes and bones, rhinitis, rashes and deformities of the teeth.

The spirochaete responsible for syphilis can only develop in human beings. Since, in Western countries, cases are nowadays treated early and successfully, it is becoming uncommon. But it still occurs quite frequently in the Far East and in parts of Central and South America.

Diagnosis: The spirochaete can be easily seen by darkground microscopy in fluid obtained from the primary chancre. It cannot be cultivated. In secondary and tertiary syphilis diagnosis depends on the demonstration of antibodies in the circulating blood by the *Treponema pallidum* haemagglutination and fluorescent treponemal antibody tests (T.P.H.A. & F.T.A. tests).

Treatment: Penicillin.

Preventive measures: Avoidance of sexual intercourse with individuals known to be or likely to be infected. Early and persistent treatment of all cases to eliminate the reservoir of infection.

2. The yaws spirochaete

Treponema pertenue

This organism is indistinguishable from the spirochaete of syphilis.

It causes *yaws*, an infection of the skin particularly common in tropical countries. It occurs chiefly in children and results in the formation of nodular ulcers. It is acquired by personal contact and its transmission is greatly facilitated by dirt, poverty, etc. It is not a veneral infection.

Diagnosis: The spirochaete, which cannot be cultivated, can be demonstrated by dark-ground microscopy, in preparations from the lesions. The T.P.H.A. and F.T.A. tests are positive.

Treatment: Penicillin.

Preventive measures: Improvement in the standard of living, attention to hygiene and the treatment of known cases with penicillin.

3. The pinta spirochaete

Treponema pinta

This organism is indistinguishable from the spirochaete of syphilis.

It causes *pinta*, a non-veneral infection characterized by skin lesions. It is prevalent in the West Indies and Central America.

Diagnosis: Consists in demonstrating the spirochaete in the lesions by dark-ground microscopy.

Treatment: Penicillin.

Preventive measures: Attention to hygiene and raising the standard of living.

4. The Vincent's angina spirochaete

Borrelia vincenti

This organism possesses much more open spirals than that responsible for syphilis.

It produces the disease known as *Vincent's angina or trench mouth* in which there is inflammation and ulceration of the fauces, gums and mucous membrane of the mouth. There is also sore throat, slight fever, and enlargement of the glands in the neck. Recovery usually occurs. In many cases fusiform bacilli are present.

Diagnosis: Examination of stained films from the lesions will reveal the presence of the spiral organisms together with the pointed rods of *Bacteroides*.

Treatment: Penicillin.
Preventive measures: Other than general hygienic measures, there are none.

5. The relapsing fever spirochaetes

Borrelia recurrentis; Borrelia duttoni

These organisms grow in the form of open spirals and are motile.

Both produce the disease known as *relapsing fever* in which they are injected into the skin by a biting insect and after an incubation period of 5 to 7 days, reach the blood stream to produce severe symptoms in the form of rigors, headache, sweats, pains over the long bones and enlargement of the spleen. The temperature reaches 103 °F or 104 °F and may persist for 5 to 7 days when it falls abruptly.

An apyrexial period of about 6 days then follows succeeded by a relapse in which signs and symptoms develop somewhat similar to those seen in the initial attack. The temperature falls after pyrexia lasting about a week when convalescence usually sets in; but more relapses occasionally occur.

Borrelia recurrentis is found in Eastern Europe where it is transmitted by lice, whereas *Borrelia duttoni* occurs in Africa and is transmitted by ticks.

Diagnosis: The spirochaetes can be seen in enormous numbers in stained films of the blood taken during the febrile periods.

Treatment: Penicillin.
Preventive measures: Insect eradication by delousing or the use of insecticides.

6. The leptospirosis spirochaetes

Leptospira icterohaemorrhagiae, etc.

These organisms are all tightly wound spirals with hooked ends which gives them the appearance of a walking stick. They are actively motile.

Several different species can cause infection in human beings but *Leptospira icterohaemorrhagiae* is responsible for most of the cases in Great Britain. They all produce the disease known as *leptospirosis* or *Weil's disease*. The onset is usually sudden with pyrexia, vomiting and marked prostration. The symptoms are, for the most part, due to infection of the liver. It becomes tender and enlarged and jaundice results in about half the cases. In some infections, there may be meningitis and haemorrhages into the skin. The illness usually lasts three to five weeks when recovery occurs in most of the cases.

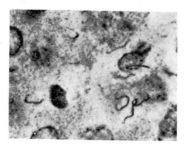

Fig. 12.1 Spirochaete of leptospirosis.

The organisms are invariably derived from an animal. The rat is the most important because it may harbour the spirochaetes for long periods and excrete them in the urine. In this way, they reach water and are conveyed to human beings who drink it. But they can also get into cuts or scratches. It is because of this that people whose work brings them into contact with rats, such as sewer workers or miners, are particularly liable to contract the disease.

Another species, *Leptospira canicola*, may come from dogs and produce very much the same symptoms in human beings. Still other species produce the disease in the Far East and Australia where the disease is much commoner than in Great Britain.

Diagnosis: The organisms can be seen by dark-ground microscopy of the blood. They will also grow in suitable culture media and can be isolated in this way from both blood and urine. They will infect young guinea pigs if the blood or urine is injected into the peritoneum. This produces jaundice, with subcutaneous and other haemorrhages.

Antibodies that can agglutinate cultures of the leptospira appear in the circulating blood during the second week of the illness.

Treatment: Penicillin if given early.

Preventive measures: Eradication of rats; preventing them from reaching drinking water, bathing pools and abattoirs. In tropical countries, avoidance of walking barefoot and attention to hygiene in dairy farms. Care in handling of patients and wearing of gloves when dealing with urine or catheterizing patients whose urine is infected.

13

The mycoplasmas, rickettsiae and chlamydiae

Although all these organisms are bacteria they have rather different properties from the bacteria previously described.
A. The Mycoplasmas
B. The Rickettsiae
C. The Chlamydiae

A. THE MYCOPLASMAS

Mycoplasma pneumoniae

These organisms do not possess properly developed cell walls and for this reason may not assume any particular shape. They are responsible for a number of serious infections in animals. The only human disease caused by them is a form of *pneumonia* previously known—but incorrectly—as virus pneumonia.

The incubation period appears to be about three weeks, but in many cases subclinical infection only is produced. If there are symptoms, they consist of a remittent fever lasting about 10 days with a dry cough and widespread radiological changes in the lungs. Secondary infection by bacteria, particularly staphylococci may also occur.

202

Diagnosis: This is usually done by demonstrating the presence of antibodies in the patient's serum. The organisms are difficult to isolate. It is however possible to cultivate them on suitable media. They form minute almost invisible colonies on solid media.

Treatment: Tetracyclines.

Preventive measures: None.

B. THE RICKETTSIAE

These organisms are minute coccobacilli just large enough to be visible on microscopic examination.

1. The typhus fever rickettsiae

Rickettsia prowazeki, Rickettsia mooseri, Rickettsia tsutsugamushi, Rickettsia typhi

They produce the disease known as *typhus* which is generally an acute febrile infection with an accompanying rash consisting of dull red blotches with a somewhat indefinite border. Severe headache is usual with delirium and death in 10–20 per cent of the cases.

The sources from which the organisms come and the methods by which they reach human beings vary with the species of rickettsiae responsible but all of them are insect-borne diseases. Thus, the rickettsiae of *epidemic typhus* are human organisms transmitted from person to person by lice. In *endemic typhus*, they come from rats and are conveyed by fleas. In *scrub typhus*, they come from small mammals and are transported by mites, but in *Rocky Mountain spotted fever* they are derived from larger wild mammals and are conveyed to human beings by ticks.

Because of its method of transmission, epidemic typhus is particularly liable to occur in wartime or during social upheavals when there is overcrowding, poverty and a lack of facilities for bathing or the washing of clothes.

Diagnosis: The organisms are generally present in the circulating blood and infect guinea pigs if injected into the groin. This is usually detected by a rise in temperature after an interval of 8–14 days.

A second and much simpler method is the Weil-Felix reaction. In this, the serum of the patient is mixed with a suspension of special strains of *Proteus vulgaris*. Agglutination occurs if the patient has typhus. This test becomes positive about the seventh day of the illness.

Treatment: Tetracyclines.

Preventive measures: Eradiciation of lice and mites by insecticides. For the prevention of epidemic and endemic typhus prophylactic immunization with a vaccine of killed rickettsiae which have been grown in eggs.

2. The Q fever rickettsia

Coxiella burneti

This organism causes *Q fever* (or *Query fever*). It is a form of atypical pneumonia.

The organism is a parasite of animals such as cows and sheep, and may reach human beings by ticks, mites or milk.

Diagnosis: Although the organism is present in the blood and will infect guinea pigs if injected into the peritoneum, diagnosis usually depends on showing that antibodies capable of reacting with the organism have appeared during the illness.

Treatment: Tetracyclines.

Preventive measures: Pasteurization of milk.

C. THE CHLAMYDIAE

These organisms are spheres just large enough to be visible with the optical microscope. They cause three human diseases.

1. The trachoma organism

Chlamydia trachomatis

These organisms infect the eye causing three types of disease known as *punctate keratitis, inclusion conjunctivitis* and *trachoma* of which the third is by far the most important. It is a chronic inflammatory condition of the eyelids, common in

North Africa, Egypt and the Near East. It is generally acquired in childhood as a result of contact with other cases or transport of the organism by house flies or communal articles such as towels. After an incubation period of five to seven days, inflammatory changes appear on the upper part of the conjunctiva. There is also a muco-purulent exudate due to secondary infection. This acute stage of the disease usually subsides but is followed by chronic inflammation which leads to scarring of the conjunctiva and cornea. Bacterial infection of the inflamed area may increase the severity of the condition. This leads to such marked deformity of the eyes and eyelids that the patient becomes partially or even completely blind.

Chlamydia trachomatis is also responsible for some cases of non-specific urethritis and the genital tract of the mother is the source of infection for reonatal conjunctivitis

Diagnosis: In smears from the eyelids stained with Giemsa there may be cells containing inclusion bodies which in fact consist of large numbers of the organisms.

Treatment: Tetracyclines.

Preventive measures: Trachoma Eradication of flies; personal cleanliness, particularly of the faces of children, to discourage flies. Communal towels, should not be used. Care on the part of nurses to wash hands after attending cases.

Non-specific urethritis As for other venereal diseases.

2. The lymphogranuloma organism

Infection by this organism is a *veneral disease* which is rare in Great Britain but relatively common in America and the coastal areas of certain tropical countries. The primary lesion is a vesicle that soon bursts to form an ulcer. This heals but is followed by enlargement of the lymph glands. They may suppurate and if this occurs in the pelvis the resulting fibrosis may cause stricture of the rectum or a form of elephantiasis.

Diagnosis: Although the organism can be isolated in eggs or in mice, the disease is usually diagnosed by the Frei test. In this, a suspension of the oreanisms, killed by heat, is injected into the skin of the patient. If an area of induration and erythema develops, it is probable that the patient is infected by the organism.

Treatment: Tetracyclines.
Preventive measures: Same as for all venereal diseases.

3. The psittacosis organism

Chlamydia psittaci

This organism produces *psittacosis*, a form of interstitial pheu-
monia usually acquired as a result of contact with birds such
as parrots, budgerigars and pigeons who may faecal carriers.
   Diagnosis: The organism is present in the sputum and produces infection in mice if injected intraperitoneally. A rise in
antibody level occurs.
   Treatment: Tetracyclines.
   Preventive measures: Prohibition of the importation of
parrots. Cleanliness in aviaries.

The fungi and actinomyces

Although the actinomyces are bacteria they can be considered with the fungi as they have some properties in common.

A. THE FUNGI

Fungi cause many diseases in human beings. Most of them are unknown in Great Britain although some such as *histoplasmosis*, *torulosis* and *blastomycosis* occur, but so rarely that it is unnecessary to say more about them. On the other hand, *ringworm*, *tinea pedis* and *thrush* are comparatively common.

1. The dermatophyle fungi

Microsporum audouini, Trichophyton mentagrophytes, etc.

These fungi grow in the form of long filaments called hyphae. They also produce bodies of varying sizes called arthrospores, conidia and chlamydospores, particularly when growing in culture.

They can only infect tissues containing keratin because they require it as a foodstuff and for this reason confine their activities to the hair, skin and nails, the only parts of the body containing this substance. When growing in the hair, they produce ringworm. The hair fractures, not far from the skin, and the distal portion falls off leaving a partially bald area.

The skin over most of the body is apparently resistant but fungi can multiply in the webs between the toes and produce *tinea pedis* or *athlete's foot*. Vesicles form which soon rupture leaving an itching, raw, ulcerated area.

The *nails* are only seldom infected but if it occurs, they become brittle, friable, opaque and discoloured.

In many instances the organisms are derived from other human beings but some species of fungi may come from cattle, cats or dogs.

Diagnosis: In ringworm, this generally involves microscopic examination of the infected hairs and in tinea pedis, scales from the skin. After clearing by soaking in 10 per cent potassium hydroxide, the characteristic hyphae and spores can generally be seen quite easily. It is usually unnecessary to cultivate the fungi but if required they grow easily on special media.

Treatment: Removal of hairs and oral griseofulvin.

Preventive measures: Isolation of cases of ringworm or at least, removal from school; destruction of cats or other household pets if suspected of being the source; and the use of antiseptics to prevent infection of the feet in communal baths.

2. Candida

Candida albicans

This fungus grows in the form of very large, pointed oval cells.

This organism is mainly responsible for thrush an infection of the mouth and fauces which usually occurs in marasmic infants but sometimes in adults debilitated by some wasting disease. It may also occur as a complication of antibiotic therapy probably because the ordinary commensals in the mouth and gut are killed, leaving a clear field for the growth of the fungus which is not susceptible to the ordinary antibiotics. This organism may also produce an infection of the vulva and vagina, sometimes but not invariably associated with pregnancy.

Diagnosis: The organisms can generally be seen in stained films from the lesions. They can also be cultivated without difficulty.

Treatment: Nystatin.

Preventive measures: None other than oral hygiene.

B. ACTINOMYCES

Actinomyces israelii

This organism grows in the form of long thin threads. *Actinomycosis* is a chronic inflammatory condition of the tissues in the neighbourhood of the alimentary canal or of the lung.

Diagnosis: Pus from the lesions contains yellow granules about the size of a pin's head and if these are crushed and stained they will be seen to consist of tangled masses of long threads. The organism will grow on artificial media provided oxygen be excluded.

Treatment: Penicillin.

Preventive measures: None.

15

The viruses

Viruses can multiply only in living cells and they differ in a number of ways from the micro-organisms described so far. They cause many of the very common infections of man.

A. Poxviruses
B. Myxoviruses
C. Togaviruses
D. Enteroviruses
E. Herpesviruses
F. Other viruses

A. POXVIRUSES

These viruses are too small to be seen in the optical microscope, but are known to be spherical particles about 0.0003 mm in diameter.

The smallpox virus

As smallpox had now been eradicated and the only sources of the organism is a small number of laboratories which still keep stocks of the virus no description of this disease will be given.

210

B. MYXOVIRUSES

These viruses are too small to be seen in the optical microscope, but are known to be spherical particles about 0.0001 mm in diameter.

1. The influenza virus

The incubation period of *influenza* is about 48 hours, and in typical cases, there is fever for two or three days, pains in the joints, and a considerable degree of prostration. There is usually dryness of the mucous membrane of the nose and fauces with a tendency to coughing. Bronchitis and pneumonia sometimes due to secondary invasion by organisms such as staphylococci are by no means rare. Convalescence is usually prolonged.

The disease occurs generally in the form of epidemics every two years, which spread rapidly from country to country along the usual lines of communication. Once introduced into a semi-closed community such as a school, ship or hospital it spreads so rapidly that large numbers may be ill at the same time.

Diagnosis: The virus can usually be isolated from cases by injecting washings from the nasopharynx into tissue cultures or into the allantoic cavity of the developing egg. A second method of diagnosis is to demonstrate an increase in the antibody level of the circulating blood during the illness by comparing specimens of blood taken during the acute and convalescent phases of the illness.

Treatment: None.

Preventive measures: An inactivated vaccine is available but its value is still doubtful.

2. The mumps virus

This virus is the same size as that of influenza. The incubation period of *mumps* is 18–21 days following which the parotid glands swell and swallowing is painful. Occasionally there may be involvement of the sub-maxillary and sub-lingual glands. The acute symptoms last for about a week following which recovery is usually rapid. In adults there is a marked tendency to complications in the form of *orchitis* and *epididymitis* in the male and inflammation of the ovary in the female. These may not only be extremely painful manifestations, but prolong the illness considerably. *Pancreatitis* and *encephalitis* may also occur.

The disease spreads from person to person probably by the saliva and enters the gland by the parotid duct.

Diagnosis: This is usually unnecessary but if essential, the virus may be isolated from saliva or throat washings. Detection of a rise in the antibody level during the illness may also be employed.

Treatment: None.

Preventive measures: None other than isolation of cases.

3. The measles virus

After an incubation period of 9–17 days the prodromal stage of *measles* sets in. This is characterized by pyrexia, catarrhal symptoms and the presence of Koplik's spots on the mucous membrane inside the cheeks. The typical rash then appears. Recovery is usual but broncho-pneumonia due to secondary infection by bacteria may occur.

Measles is probably spread by the nasopharyngeal secretions during the prodromal stage.

Diagnosis: On clinical grounds only.

Treatment: Antibiotics when pneumonia occurs.

Preventive measures: Isolation of cases. Human gamma globulin can be employed to give passive protection if necessary. As the patient is infective before the appearance of the rash nothing much can be done in the way of prevention, but as far as possible young and debilitated children should be kept away from a child suffering from measles. A vaccine made from a living attenuated strain of the virus is available, and routine immunization is recommended.

4. The rabies virus

Rabies is a disease of dogs and related species such as wolves, coyotes, jackals and foxes. It may however occur in other animals such as skunks, rabbits and vampire bats. Human beings acquire rabies as a result of a bite by an animal in the acute stage of the disease.

The incubation period may vary from a few days to several months following which the patient becomes extremely ill with symptoms of acute cerebral excitement. A prominent feature of the disease is inability to swallow. This phase of the disease gradually merges into a paralytic phase. Death is the invariable ending and may occur in either phase of the disease.

The disease has become common amongst the foxes of France and is gradually approaching the Channel coast with the possibility that it may become endemic in England. For this reason heavy penalties are now imposed for the importation of pets such as dogs, cats and other domestic animals that have not been subjected to quarantine for six months.

Diagnosis: Entirely clinical. But the fact that the patient has rabies can be confirmed by examination of the brain of the animal from which he acquired the disease. Microscopic examination may reveal the presence of minute collections of the virus in certain cells. These are known as Negri bodies.

Treatment: None.

Preventive measures: Quarantine for 6 months of all dogs entering countries free of the disease. Prophylactic immunization of dogs with vaccine. Active immunization of human beings who have been bitten, and passive immunization with serum containing antibodies for the virus.

C. TOGAVIRUSES

Referred to in previous editions as Arboviruses, these viruses are all very small spheres only 0.00003 to 0.00004 mm in diameter. They are derived from members of the animal kingdom and are transmitted by arthropod insects.

1. The yellow fever virus

Yellow fever makes its appearance after an incubation period of 3–4 days. The onset is sudden with fever, headache and backache. Nausea and vomiting are usual. In 3–4 days the temperature may fall, only to rise again. It is during this period that the jaundice appears which gives the disease its name. There is a marked tendency to bleeding, particularly from the gums. Vomiting, the vomitus containing blood—the so-called 'black vomit'—may also occur. A high proportion of cases are fatal, death usually occurring on the sixth or seventh day.

Basically, yellow fever is a disease of the monkey population of certain tropical countries such as South and Central America and Central Africa, but can be conveyed from the monkeys to human beings by mosquitoes. Once this has occurred it can be then transmitted from human being to human being by a domesticated species of mosquitoes known as *Aedes aegypti*. Largely because it can only be transmitted by mosquitoes, it is limited in distribution to those countries where the climate is suitable for their development. For this reason, the disease is largely confined to Central Africa and the northern part of South America (see Fig. 7.2).

Diagnosis: Mice become infected by the virus if blood from patients taken before the fifth day of the illness be injected into the brain.

Treatment: None.

Preventive measures: Prophylactic immunization with a living but attenuated strain of the virus. Eradication of the insect vector by drainage of marshes and standing water, by surface application of paraffin oil, or by spraying with a larvicide such as arsenic. Screening of houses and spraying with insecticides. International methods include spraying with insecticides aircraft coming from the endemic areas.

2. The dengue virus

Dengue comes on after an incubation period of 5–9 days. The resulting illness resembles a severe attack of influenza, with pyrexia lasting for 6–7 days, headache, backache and pain in the joints of sufficient severity to warrant the name, 'break-bones fever'. A maculopapular or scarlatiniform rash may appear on the third, fourth or fifth day and lasts 3–4 days. Death from dengue is rare and mild cases are not unusual.

In many respects dengue resembles yellow fever in that its true home is the monkey population of tropical countries, but once it has been transferred to man it can be transmitted from person to person by *Aedes aegypti* mosquitoes. Many quite severe epidemics have been produced in this way. It is, therefore, limited in distribution to countries where these mosquitoes can breed, that is to say, Greece and the neighbouring countries, the southern United States and Central America, northern Australia and Japan.

Diagnosis: Since it is difficult to isolate the virus, this procedure is of little value. But a retrospective diagnosis may be obtained if the antibody level in the circulating blood rises during the illness. This may be detected by taking samples of blood as early as possible in the disease and another when recovery has occurred. The antibody level in the two samples can be estimated by the complement fixation test.

Treatment: None.

Preventive measures: Anti-mosquito methods such as screens for windows, mosquito netting for beds and insect-repellent creams.

3. The sandfly fever virus

Sandfly fever resembles influenza. After an incubation period of 2–6 days, there is a sudden rise in temperature which persists for 2–4 days.

The disease is limited in distribution to the Mediterranean and the Black Sea, the Near East and the contiguous parts of India and the U.S.S.R. So far as is known, there is no animal reservoir of this virus; only human beings are infected by it. On the coast of the Adriatic, it is trasmitted by female midges known as pappatici or *Phlebotomus papatasi*.

Diagnosis: Rise in antibody level during the illness.

Treatment: None.

Preventive measures: Measures for the eradication of insects, particularly spraying of floors and crevices in brickwork, etc., with insecticides.

4. The encephalitis viruses

Many different viruses can produce encephalitis in addition to their more usual activities. Encephalitis may, therefore, occur as a complication in mumps and measles, to name only two instances. But many viruses are now known whose only pathological activity so fat as human beings are concerned is the production of encephalitis.

The symptoms are indicative of damage to the brain, but vary too much in type and severity to enable a summary to be made. It is however of considerable importance that whenever the disease makes its appearance, many other individuals are evidently infected by the virus without showing signs and symptoms. Indeed subclinical infections generally outnumber the actual cases.

The viruses responsible are all fundamentally pathogens of birds or mammals. A second peculiarity is that almost without exception they are carried to human beings by arthropod insects such as mosquitoes, mites, ticks, etc. On the whole, these viruses are commoner in tropical or subtropical countries than in temperate climates. Indeed the only form of encephalitis due to an organism in this group that occurs in this country is *benign lymphocytic meningitis*. But in Australia for example, there is *Murray Valley encephalitis, St. Louis encephalitis* in North America and *Japanese B encephalitis* in the Far East, while a whole series of different viruses are responsible for encephalitis in Africa and South America.

Diagnosis: The virus can only be isolated if the patient dies because it is necessary to inject a suspension of the brain into the brains of mice. If the patient recovers, the diagnosis rests on the demonstration of a rise in antibody level for the virus. This necessitates comparison between blood samples taken during the acute phase of the illness and a second during convalescence.

Treatment: None.

Preventive measures: Eradication of the insect responsible for carrying the infection.

D. ENTEROVIRUSES

The viruses in this group are very small spherical particles about 0.00003 mm in diameter. They are all primarily parasites of the human intestinal tract but may reach other organs to produce characteristic syndromes.

1. The poliomyelitis virus

The incubation period of *poliomyelitis* is not known with certainty but varies from 5–35 days, although the majority of cases first show symptoms 7–14 days after exposure. The clinical picture varies enormously. The majority of those harbouring the virus during an epidemic do not suffer from any definite involvement of the central nervous system. Their symptoms resemble those of influenza or the derangements of the gastrointestinal tract usually associated with food infections. In a minority of cases, however, the virus reaches the central nervous system where it attacks the motor nerve cells in the cord and medulla to produce paralytic poliomyelitis. It has been calculated that as a general rule only one case out of every hundred harbouring the virus during epidemic periods shows symptoms of paralysis.

In the course of growth in the motor nerve cells, necrosis is produced so that they no longer control the groups of muscles to which they are connected. This produces paralysis which is generally permanent. The number of cells attacked in this way and the extent of the resulting paralysis vary greatly, but the most important feature of this process is the danger that the muscles of respiration may be affected. This is usually the cause of death. The cerebrum and cerebellum are not as a rule attacked.

It is probable that the main reservoir from which the virus comes is the human population of tropical or subtropical countries in the Mediterranean littoral, the Philippines, Central America, and probably other areas as well. There it reaches practically every child before its fifth birthday. The great majority suffer from inapparent or subclinical infection and only a very small minority show symptoms of paralysis. Although the virus may reach countries with temperate climates, widespread immunization against the disease has resulted in clinically apparent infection becoming extremely unusual.

Convalescents from the disease and a high proportion of those in contact with patients may have the virus in the stools for comparatively long periods. It is probable that transfer of the organism from the stools to food is the method by which the disease is transmitted.

Diagnosis: This usually consists in demonstrating the presence of the virus in the stools by inoculating them into tissue cultures. A rise in antibody level during the illness may also be employed.

Treatment: None.

Preventive measures: Isolation or barrier nursing of cases. Prophylactic immunization with a living vaccine made from growth of virus in tissue cultures which is administered by mouth.

2. The Coxsackie virus

This virus is named after the village in New York State in which it was first found. It produces three syndromes.

Bornholm disease, sometimes known as *epidemic myalgia* or *pleurodynia*, generally occurs in the form of small epidemics. The incubation period varies from 2–9 days, following which there is an abrupt onset with fever and acute pain, usually in the thoracic or abdominal regions. Recovery occurs after an illness lasting only a few days or as much as 2 weeks.

A second manifestation is *acute herpangina*, which is a febrile illness lasting from 1–14 days, with sore throat due to the development of discrete vesicular lesions on the anterior pillars of the fauces, but less often on other areas of the pharynx. The disease tends to occur in epidemic form in young children during the summer months.

Aseptic meningitis with fever, headache and abdominal pains and signs of meningeal irritation may also be caused by viruses of this group. Recovery is the rule.

The virus is present in the stools, and is probably conveyed by food or water. It is frequently present in normal individuals who have no sign of illness whatever.

Diagnosis: The virus may be isolated from the stools by tissue culture methods. A rise in antibody level of the blood for the virus can also be employed.

Treatment: None.

Preventive measures: None, other than care over the disposal of the faeces of cases.

3. The echo viruses

Entero-cytopathogenic-human-orphan viruses

These viruses produce several different syndromes in human beings; (1) *fever with rhinorrhoea*, (2) *diarrhoea* with or without a rash, and (3) *aseptic meningitis.* Many of these viruses may be present in the stools of normal people who have no symptoms of any kind.

They are probably transmitted as a result of facal contamination of food or water.

Diagnosis: These viruses may be isolated by tissue culture methods from the throat and faeces; and in cases with meningitis, from the cerebrospinal fluid.

Treatment: None.

Preventive measures: None.

4. The common cold virus

Common colds are so well known that it is hardly necessary to describe them. But many of the later symptoms are undoubtedly due to secondary bacterial invasion of the mucous membrane by bacteria in the respiratory tract.

It is certain that these infections are due to viruses but very little is as yet known about those that are probably responsible. It would seem however that colds may be due to infection by several viruses.

Diagnosis: The viruses may be isolated from nasal secretions or throat washings inoculated into tissue cultures.

Treatment: None.

Preventive measures: None.

E. HERPESVIRUSES

There are four viruses in this group.

1. The chickenpox and herpes zoster virus

One virus produces both diseases but the symptoms and way in which they are caused are very different. *Chickenpox* or

Varicella is usually acquired in childhood as a result of contact with another case of the disease. The incubation period is 14–16 days following which there is fever and, about 24 hours later, the development of the rash which consists of papules which develop into vesicles and pustules; crusts then develop over the pustules. The rash superficially resembles that of mild smallpox but there are important differences in its distribution and severity.

Herpes Zoster or *Shingles* on the other hand, generally occur in older persons and the symptoms are due to growth of the virus in the dorsal nerve roots and the nerves connected therewith. As a result there is an extremely painful eruption on the skin over the area of distribution of the nerve. The eruption takes the form of vesicles. Except for the danger to the eye when the fifth cranial nerve is involved, the condition eventually clears up, but some patients have severe post herpetic neuralgia. The disease is due to re-activation of the virus which has remained dormant in the dorsal nerve roots for many years.

Diagnosis: A rise in antibody level using the complement fixation test may be demonstrated.

Treatment: Unnecessary in chickenpox but when herpes zoster threatens to invade the eye, treatment with idoxuridine may be required.

Preventive measures: None.

2. Herpes simplex virus

Herpes simplex is a vesicular eruption of the skin or mucous membrane usually in the region of the mouth or nose. It commonly occurs as a complication of colds, influenza or prolonged exposure to sunlight or cold. In children a more extensive eruption such as *aphthous stomatitis* or *Kaposis' varicelliform eruption* may also be due to this virus.

Diagnosis: The virus will infect animals, developing eggs or tissue cultures.

Treatment: Idoxuridine.

Preventive measures: None.

3. Cytomegalovirus

So-called because it tends to produce greatly enlarged cells in the tissues. This virus usually produces a symptomless infection in a high proportion of the human race. But it may cause a severe disease in young children in which there are *haemolytic anaemia, jaundice* and enlargement of the *liver* and *spleen*. The lungs and central nervous system may also be invaded. Even if recovery occurs, *mental retardation* and *muscular disability* may result. *Congenital infection* before birth may also occur with somewhat similar symptoms appearing when the child is born.

Diagnosis: In general, this is not possible but the virus may be isolated from the urine or throat using tissue cultures.

Treatment: None.

Preventive measures: None.

4. Epstein Barr virus

There is an association between this virus and the tumours of Burkitt's lymphoma. It is also a cause of glandular fever (infectious mononucleosis).

F. OTHER VIRUSES

1. The infective hepatitis virus

Since this virus does not infect animals or grow in tissue cultures, very little is known about the appearance or general properties of this virus.

It produces *infective hepatitis* usually in the form of small epidemics. The liver is the principal organ involved accompanied by jaundice in about half the cases. The incubation period varies from 10–40 days but is usually 21–25 days. The symptoms comprise a vague feeling of illness, muscular weakness and abdominal discomfort, accompanied by vomiting and pyrexia.

The virus is present in the stools and is probably conveyed to others in food and water.

Diagnosis: On clinical grounds only.

Treatment: None.

Preventive measures: Care in handling excreta. Prophylactic administration of normal immunoglobulin for contacts.

2. The serum hepatitis virus

Clinically, *serum hepatitis* or *Type B hepatitis* closely resembles infective hepatitis but may be more severe with a higher death rate. The incubation period is even longer being 60–120 days. Its causation is also very different. It is conveyed from person to person by blood from symptomless carriers of the virus. It may therefore, follow blood tranfusions or injections with syringes contaiminated by the blood of other persons. It can also be conveyed to those handling the apparatus employed for renal dialysis.

Diagnosis: Detection of the so-called Australia antigen in the blood.

Treatment: None.

Preventive measures: Care that blood from one person does not reach others when hypodermic injections are being given and that blood from donors who are Australia antigen positive is not used for transfusions. Passive immunization may be given to people with a high risk of infection.

3. The rubella virus

The incubation period of *rubella* or *german measles* is 14–21 days when pyrexia with conjunctivitis, headache and dryness of the throat appear at about the same time as the rash which consists of rose pink spots somewhat resembling the rash of scarlet fever in colour. Enlargement of the occipital glands also occurs.

The particular importance of german measles is that if it occurs during the first 3 months of pregnancy, the foetus may be so affected that it may exhibit certain stigmata at birth or which develop some time later. These include microcephaly, deaf mutism, congenital heart defects, cataract and mental retardation.

Diagnosis A rise in antibody level during the disease.

Treatment: None.

Preventive measures: Pregnant women should avoid contact with the disease. A vaccine is now available and should be given to girls before puberty.

4. The adenoviruses

These viruses infect the cells of the respiratory tract or the eye and cause six different syndromes: (1) an acute febrile *pharyngitis*; (2) a febrile infection of the *respiratory tract* resembling a cold; (3) febrile *pharyngitis* with *conjunctivitis*; (4) *primary atypical pneumonia*; (5) acute follicular *conjunctivitis* and (6) epidemic *kerato-conjunctivitis.*

It is unnecessary to describe each syndrome in detail but there seems to be no doubt that they are due to transfer from person to person of tears or secretions from the nasopharynx.

Diagnosis: All the viruses responsible will multiply in the cells of tissue cultures.

Treatment: None.

Preventive measures: In general, none but epidemic kerato-conjunctivitis has been shown to be transmissible in the eye clinics by eye droppers so that a technique must be adopted which prevents this.

5. Marburg virus

Given this name because the disease was first detected in the city of Marburg in Germany, it is now known to be a natural parasite of vervet monkeys in central Africa.

After an incubation period of 3–9 days, the symptoms produced comprise, high fever, myalgia, vomiting, diarrhoea, hepatitis, a maculopapular rash with a marked tendency to bleeding. The symptoms are severe and a fatal ending not uncommon. It should also be mentioned that the disease may be highly infectious.

Diagnosis: The clinical picture is characteristic. The virus may be isolated in laboratory animals.

Treatment: None.

Preventive measures: Strict isolation of infected patients. Care in the handling of monkeys.

6. Lassa fever

The virus responsible is a parasite of a small rodent *Mastomyces natalensis* in central Africa and is excreted in the urine.

This is probably the source of human infections. These are often mild but the more severe cases have high fever, sore throat, vomiting, abdominal and chest pains with marked prostration. Recovery may occur but the condition of the patient may deteriorate with serous effusions, oedema and haemorrhages which lead to death. The disease is easily trasmitted by the urine, faeces, vomit or saliva.

Diagnosis: The virus will multiply in tissue culture and may be isolated from urine and from the throat.

Treatment: None.

Preventive measures: Very strict isolation of the infected patients.

7. Rotavirus

This name is given because of the characteristic wheel like appearance when examined by electron microscopy. They are a cause of diarrhoea in babies.

Diagnosis: Demonstration of the particles by electron microscopy.

Treatment: General supportive measures.

Preventive measures: Isolation of infected babies.

Index

225